GINGER
COMMON SPICE & WONDER DRUG

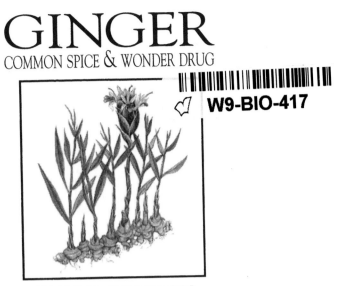

THIRD EDITION

GINGER
COMMON SPICE & WONDER DRUG

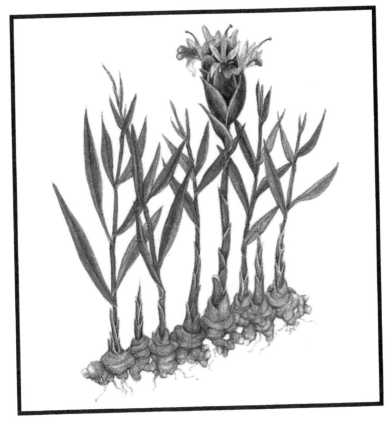

THIRD EDITION

Paul Schulick

Kalindi Press

THIRD EDITION

Copyright © 2012 by Paul Schulick

Cover and text design by Sally Nichols
Cover illustration by Kay Life
Back cover photo by Alan Gill

Previous editions copyrighted in 1993 and 1994

Kalindi Press
P.O. Box 4410
Chino Valley, AZ 86323
800-381-2700
www.kalindipress.com, hppublisher@cableone.net

Author's Note:

As remarkable and promising as the research on ginger is, it is important for the reader to recognize that there is no herb that can replace the value of exercise, good diet, a healthy environment or a contented state of mind.

It is also critical that the reader understand that ginger cannot replace the expertise of a highly trained holistic health practitioner. Readers should consult with their practitioner before adopting the therapeutic applications in this book.

The author and publishers disclaim any liability arising directly or indirectly from the use of this book.

CONTENTS

FIGURES

Thanks and Tribute

My thanks to . . .

Dr. K.C. Srivastava for his guidance and years of research on ginger and eicosanoids.

Mary Lou Quinn and Dr. Norman Farnsworth and all those who have worked on the Napralert project, the world's most complete database on natural remedies.

My wife, Barbi Schulick, for her invaluable editing and support and my two children, Geremy and Rosalie, for keeping my life in perspective.

Barbara Grenquist for her editorial skills.

Sally Nichols for her attention and care in bringing the text of this book to life.

All those who work on the shared vision to restore natural remedies to their rightful place.

My tribute to . . .

The millions of animals who have paid a price with their lives and suffering in the name of human protection. I pay tribute to their sacrifice and pray that it is not in vain. I look forward to a day when animal testing is no longer deemed necessary and alternatives are found.

1
FROM THE START

Beyond Sisyphus

In Greek mythology, Sisyphus, a king of Corinth, was condemned forever to roll a huge stone up a hill in Hades only to have it roll down again on nearing the top.

❧NOTE❧

Why is it necessary in a book on ginger to question the priorities of medical education, to detail the costs of marketing a drug or expose the underlying philosophy of the food industry? Forces are at play within these conditions that will ultimately determine the fate of whatever promise ginger happens to hold. This chapter alerts the reader to grave threats to our health freedom while offering a vision of hope. In the last chapter, "Freedom and Health at the Crossroads," these issues are covered in greater depth.

Ginger, botanically known as *Zingiber officinale*, is one of the world's ten favorite spices[1] Yet, astonishingly, its most precious values are still virtually ignored or unknown. This book proposes that your spice cabinet contains a most phenomenal herb and healing entity–one that is beyond the therapeutic scope of any modern drug, with the potential to save billions of dollars and countless lives.

Is it possible that something so powerful could be ginger? If modern science can demonstrate that ordinary foods like carrots and broccoli–or even citrus mold–can offer elements (beta carotene, sulforaphane and penicillin) that can prevent disease or save millions of lives, why not a common spice? Ginger is certainly as likely to be a healing force as any of the above. It has not made its way into a majority of Oriental formulations for thousands of years by mere coincidence. Surely, every scientist would agree that a botanical like ginger *could* contain a powerful healing element since today it is estimated that at least 25 percent of all modern drugs are botanical in origin. Might we then, in our quest to isolate a single compound or drug out of its botanical context, be missing a healing miracle in the whole plant itself, especially one as readily available as ginger?

Unfortunately, over the past forty years, the prevailing health-care system and the government agencies entrusted to regulate it have virtually excluded this possibility, along with many other treatments related to so-called alternative, traditional or unorthodox medicine. Especially kept in competitive check have been herbs and other nutritional supplements, which hundreds of studies have demonstrated possess the potential to replace many modern synthesized pharmaceutical drugs.

A repression of health-care alternatives has been achieved both directly through regulatory control and indirectly through what would appear to be a systematic offensive against alternative health-care providers. For example, physicians who have recommended herbal supplements have often suffered the indignity of being labeled quacks and, more importantly, have endured the threat of financially devastating licensor losses. Few people are aware that the supplements themselves, "the tools-of-the-trade," have on occasion been seized through the use of any number of absurd technicalities. For example, the government has required that anytime a health claim about an herb or dietary supplement is made, the producers must *prove* that this supplement is a safe and effective drug.

This proving sounds fair enough, but like Sisyphus and the rock, it is a feat that is impossible to accomplish. A new drug application costs up to $359 million,[2] takes eight or more years to process and, most ironically, can never actually result in a patent because a whole herb is not a patentable substance. The only patentable item from an herb would be an isolated element, thereby excluding the value of the whole herb and the synergy or inherent cooperation this wholeness represents. So while 25 percent of all modern drugs are derived from plants, ultimately the whole plant itself is actually being ignored or discarded in favor of the one, active, patentable element. As designed, the sole purveyor who can create and sell a prescription drug to the sanctioned medical trade is our nation's most profitable corporate entity, the pharmaceutical industry.

Despite this monopolistic pressure, growing numbers of Americans are seeking out alternative forms of health care. A recent survey in the most prestigious *New England Journal of Medicine* declared that in 1990 more than one-third of all Americans had visited an alternative or unorthodox practitioner. More telling was the fact that 72 percent of these respondents who used unconventional therapy did not inform their medical doctor that they had done so.[3]

A most encouraging development is that this segment of the population has begun to organize into a politically active group. As a result of the forming of grass-roots organizations throughout the United States, alternative health as a choice can now challenge the very roots of the medical establishment and lift the rightful representation of herbs and natural health care into the current national debate on health reform. The hope is that research like this on ginger will contribute to this all-important battle for healthier choices and medical freedom.

Unless we put medical freedom into the Constitution,
the time will come when medicine will organize itself
into an undercover dictatorship. To restrict the art of
healing to doctors and deny equal privileges to others
will constitute the Bastille of medical science.
All such laws are un-American and despotic.

DR. BENJAMIN RUSH,
SIGNER OF THE DECLARATION OF INDEPENDENCE[4]

2
FROM CULTIVATION TO CONFUCIUS

ಖ಄ಖಖ

Botany 101

❧NOTE❧

Where did ginger get its name? What does ginger have in common with the principal spice in curry? What conditions are ideal for ginger cultivation, and who grows the best and the most ginger? The answers to these questions and more are a formal introduction to our favorite spice.

No one really knows the exact origins of ginger. It was probably first discovered in the tropics of Southeast Asia. Some botanists argue that its Sanskrit name indicates India as the site of origin.[1] Confirming this hypothesis, however, is next to impossible due to both secretive trade and wide cultivation which have left no documents of its origin or existence in the wild state.

Ginger was given its official botanical name, *Zingiber officinale*, by the famous eighteenth-century Swedish botanist, Linnaeus. Linnaeus derived the genus title Zingiber from its Indian Sanskrit name *singabera* which means shaped like a horn.[2]

Ginger is one of more than 1,400 species belonging to the Zingiberaceae family, sharing the family's most popular honors with the spices turmeric (a principal component of curry) and cardamom.[3] Ginger is a slender perennial reaching 24 to 39 inches in height. Its first stems are longer than the second and latter stems and bear beautifully fragrant flowers which are greenish-yellow and streaked with purple. The leaves are a dark green with a prominent midrib that is sheathed at the base, and the seeds are found in the rare fruiting body.

The most familiar part of the ginger plant used in commerce is the irregularly shaped and sized underground section which we erroneously call a root. Although ginger will probably always be associated with the term *root*, it is botanically correct to call it a rhizome. Unlike a root which dies if it is split, ginger can actually generate whole new plants from its budded sections. It is from these buds that ginger has been cultivated for thousands of years. Ginger grows best in a hot and moist climate with available shade, and in soil that is rich in loam and well tilled. The ginger rhizome is aromatic and thick lobed and ranges from white to yellow in color. One of the prized varieties and most unusual exceptions to this color range is a variety that possesses a characteristic blue ring which circles the fleshy interior.

Ginger is today the world's most widely cultivated spice. There are as many opinions as to who grows the best ginger as there are countries and regions that cultivate it. Ginger appears in so many varieties, with an estimated fifty in India alone, that any favoritism is a matter of personal taste. Each variety possesses its own distinctive flavor and aroma depending upon the soil and the manner in which it is grown. The most pungent gingers are reported to come from Africa, while milder varieties are found in China. There is some consensus that the milder gingers are better for culinary applications while the spicier varieties are best from a beverage and therapeutic standpoint. Since the focus of this book is on the medicinal properties of ginger, it is significant to note that the

only specific variety actually singled out from a therapeutic standpoint is the blue ring, which is reported to contain the highest proteolytic or protein-digesting enzyme content.[4]
(See figure 1 for the basics on growers, importers, growing conditions and harvesting.)◆

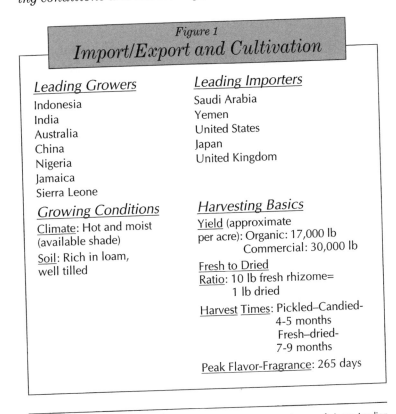

Figure 1
Import/Export and Cultivation

Leading Growers
Indonesia
India
Australia
China
Nigeria
Jamaica
Sierra Leone

Growing Conditions
Climate: Hot and moist (available shade)
Soil: Rich in loam, well tilled

Leading Importers
Saudi Arabia
Yemen
United States
Japan
United Kingdom

Harvesting Basics
Yield (approximate per acre): Organic: 17,000 lb
Commercial: 30,000 lb

Fresh to Dried Ratio: 10 lb fresh rhizome= 1 lb dried

Harvest Times: Pickled–Candied- 4-5 months
Fresh–dried- 7-9 months

Peak Flavor-Fragrance: 265 days

◆ In 1990, Indonesia led the list of growers, exporting 38,114 metric tons of ginger. Leading importers of ginger are Saudi Arabia, Yemen, the United States, Japan and the United Kingdom. In 1992, the United States imported most of its fresh ginger from Fiji, powdered from Taiwan, sweet from Hong Kong and candied from Australia.[5] Certified organic growers report that one acre of land will yield between 13,000 and 17,000 pounds of fresh ginger. Commercial yields are reported to be as high as 30,000 pounds per acre. This helps explain why prices for certified organic ginger may be as much as five times the cost of some commercial varieties.

Few spices have as wide a range of harvesting schedules as ginger. Harvesting time determines to a major extent the final form for sale; i.e., pickled, dried or fresh. As a general rule, the longer ginger is in the ground (past 5 months) the more fibrous and pungent the rhizome becomes. Therefore, when ginger is eaten straight as in the pickled or crystallized candy forms, where fiber is least desirable, it is usually harvested in 4-5 months and when ginger is used for cooking or syruping, it is harvested from 7-9 months after planting. Ginger processed for dried powders will generally be the latest in the harvesting cycle. Regardless of the final form, research suggests that ginger's flavor and fragrance constituents crest at 265 days.[6]

The Spice That Changed the World

Every good quality is contained in ginger.
AN ANCIENT INDIAN PROVERB[7]

❧NOTE❧

A book about ginger would be incomplete without some mention of its historic political impact. From its unknown botanical origin to its present status as the world's most widely cultivated spice, ginger possesses one of the herb kingdom's richest histories. Loved and defended by the likes of Confucius and King Henry VIII and lauded by Shakespeare and Islamic scripture, ginger has been a player in the creation and destruction of nations. This section details a chronological overview of ginger's worldwide movement. The medical history of ginger is addressed in the section "A Healer for 5,000 Years."

Could a common spice have helped shape modern history? Sounds like an outrageous claim, but not more than two hundred years ago spices were the political and economic equivalent of today's oil and clean water.

From the earliest written records, lucrative ginger trade routes were guarded with secrecy and intrigue. For example, early Arab traders protected their passages and personal supplies of ginger from the inquisitive and resourceful Greeks and Romans by actually fabricating a fabled land inhabited by a primitive and ruthless people they called the Troglodytes. Interestingly, the Arabs' secretive business engagements probably had more than economics at their roots. In the holiest text of Islam, the Koran, ginger is regarded as a spiritual and heavenly beverage.

Round amongst them [the righteous in Paradise] are
passed vessels of silver and goblets made of glass . . . a
cup, the admixture of which is ginger.
KORAN 76:15-17[8]

The most ancient literature of all the great civilizations of the Middle East, Asia and Europe contains testimonials to both the medicinal and economic importance of ginger. From five-thousand-year-old Greek literature to 200 B.C. Chinese records, ancient historians equated the ownership of ginger or its trade routes with prosperity. In the latter case, a Chinese historian wrote how thousands of acres were planted only in ginger and bringing immense wealth.[9] We can now understand why explorers like Marco Polo and Vasco da Gama were so careful to document the cultivation of ginger.[10]

Well into the Middle Ages, ginger sustained its economic and cultural significance. This is affirmed by records of transactions in England where just one pound was considered worth 1 shilling and 7 pence, approximately equivalent to the price of a sheep.[11] The name ginger actually became synonymous with *spice*. For hundreds of years it graced only the dinner tables of the upper class or royalty.

For thousands of years, trade in spices like ginger became the measure of an empire's wealth and power. Fortunately for ginger, its worldwide cultivation was insured by the economics of the spice trade and its stimulus to colonialism. The Spanish people, who were particularly aggressive explorers and colonialists, were one of the key nations responsible for taking ginger around the globe and encouraging its cultivation in the New World.

One might ask why ginger should have been the focus of such a historic drama. There are three principal reasons. The first and second, which will soon be discussed in depth, were a regard for ginger's powerful medicinal and food preservative properties. The third and most apparent is best expressed by Shakespeare in *Love's Labour's Lost*: "And had I but one penny in the world, thou shouldst have it to buy ginger-bread."[12]

3
THE WORKINGS OF A MIRACLE

Anatomy of a Spice

❧NOTE❧

The first step in understanding the miracle of how ginger works is to investigate its hundreds of individual parts or constituents. This is truly an awe-inspiring experience, because its components yield a virtual pharmacology course of intriguing organic compounds. The following section identifies and highlights just a few of these hundreds of elements that are at play in ginger's taste, fragrance and therapeutic effects.

Ginger's anatomy can be divided into four principal sections: 1) taste or pungency; 2) essential oil or fragrance; 3) macro/micro-nutrients; and 4) synergists.

The most obvious note of ginger's universally loved flavor is its pungency. Contained within this profoundly distinctive taste are also some of ginger's most powerful medicinal properties. The first attempt to dissect this pungency or spiciness was the work of Thresh in 1879.[1] He isolated an oily-resinous substance, comprising approximately

5 to 10 percent of the plant, and gave it the name ginerol.[2] This oleoresin has since been broken down into close to thirty elements.

The two most recognized divisions of these pungency constituents are called gingerols and shogaols. Gingerols, present in fresh ginger, convert into the more pungent shogaols with dehydration and heat. This chemical transformation from the fresh to the dry state is one of the most profound factors behind ginger's therapeutic effects. Almost as distinctive as ginger's taste is its fragrance. The wonderfully sweet, warm and citrusy aroma of ginger is highly regarded and widely used in the perfumery and beverage industries. The unique scent of ginger arises from one of nature's most complex essential oils comprising between 1.0 to 2.5 percent of the dried rhizome. After reviewing the work of more than seventeen studies, researcher Brian Lawrence[3] compiled 200 different components of this essential oil.♦ It is no wonder that V. S. Govindarajan, the author of the definitive work on the chemistry, technology and quality evaluation of ginger, concluded, "It is unlikely that the balanced aroma of natural ginger will be duplicated for a long time."[4]

The macro/micro-nutrients category encompasses proteins, lipids, carbohydrates and all the known vitamins, minerals and trace nutrients of ginger. Unlike many other herbs or spices, fresh or green ginger has a history of being consumed as a vegetable[5] and does possess considerable levels of nutrients like postassium, phosphorous, vitamin C and riboflavin (see figure 2).

Synergists are included here, with all due humility, as an escape clause to encompass the remainder of ginger's elements. Although elements like gingerols or zingiberene might be the primary constituents responsible for taste and scent respectively, many of the other hundreds of ingredients that are referred to here as synergists ultimately interact and overlap to manifest the entire effect.

♦ One of the best-known constituents of ginger oil is zingiberene, which is noted for its flavor and carminative activity.[6]

Figure 2

Nutritional Values for Fresh Ginger

Nutrient by %		Vitamins/Minerals (mg/100 gm)	
Moisture	80.9	Calcium	20.00
Protein	2.3	Phosphorous	60.00
Fat	0.9	Iron	2.60
Carbohydrates	12.3	B1	.06
Fiber	2.4	B2	.03
Minerals	1.2	B3	.60
Enzyme	2.3	C	6.00

Fresh ginger offers a full profile of nutrients. The above table is only a representative sample because there are significant variations between varieties. Nutritional values of dried ginger depend upon the reduction of moisture.[7]

Of special note in the synergists category is an enzyme called zingibain and other highly researched plant constituents like capsaicin, curcumin and limonene. Zingibain is a powerful protein-digesting enzyme that is comparable to papain from papaya and bromelain from pineapple. What is most interesting is not so much the enzyme itself but its potency. Comprising as much as 2 percent of the fresh rhizome, ginger is one of nature's richest sources of proteolytic enzymes. As a point of reference, this is approximately 180 times the amount of proteolytic enzyme contained in the papaya plant.[8] Capsaicin, curcumin and limonene are common to a number of other spices and possess a phenomenal array of physiological effects. (*See* "Ginger's Constituents and Actions" *on page 111.*)

An Infinite Cascade of Reactions

Synergy means behavior of whole systems unpredicted by
the behavior of their parts.
RICHARD BUCKMINSTER FULLER (1895-1983)[9]

✾NOTE✾

What are the mechanisms that allow ginger actually
to prevent or benefit conditions like life-threatening
heart attacks, arthritis and ulcers? Within one simple
observed effect like ginger's relief of inflammation
might be a dozen different complex chemical interactions. The sheer magnitude of these reactions leads
one seriously to question the entire paradigm of modern pharmacology, which searches for a single active
constituent. The full spectrum of ginger's actions is
probably beyond comprehension; however, understanding something about the complexity of these
mechanisms might help one better appreciate, use
and gain value from the spice.

Introduction

Ginger's observed effects are the result of an almost infinite cascade of reactions caused by literally hundreds of
individual compounds. How the more than four hundred
taste, fragrance, nutrient and synergist constituents of
ginger interact to create its profound therapeutic benefits
is an exercise in endless complexity (see figure 3).[10]

All one needs to be convinced of this intricacy is to review
the properties of its pungent taste elements. Within these
two principal groups of more than thirty constituents is a
veritable pharmacy. In an attempt to simplify and illustrate
this pharmacological dynamic, a dualistic model of principal
action and observed effect is outlined (see figure 4).

A *principal action* is defined here as the consequence
of the combining of one or more active or inactive con-

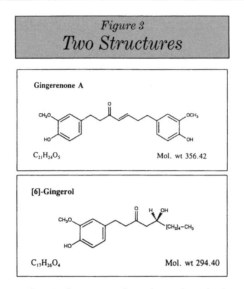

Figure 3
Two Structures

Gingerenone A

$C_{21}H_{24}O_5$ Mol. wt 356.42

[6]-Gingerol

$C_{17}H_{26}O_4$ Mol. wt 294.40

Chemical structures have been described for literally hundreds of the constituents of ginger. The above structures are included as examples of two with defined physiological activities.[11]

stituents. Through these bonds or interactions, the original activity of one constituent is intensified, modified or negated. A principal action either alone or more typically

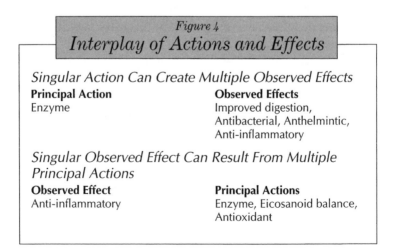

Figure 4
Interplay of Actions and Effects

Singular Action Can Create Multiple Observed Effects

Principal Action	Observed Effects
Enzyme	Improved digestion, Antibacterial, Anthelmintic, Anti-inflammatory

Singular Observed Effect Can Result From Multiple Principal Actions

Observed Effect	Principal Actions
Anti-inflammatory	Enzyme, Eicosanoid balance, Antioxidant

in association with other principal actions will then result in a myriad of observed effects. As shown in figure 4, an observed effect can easily have at its roots a variety of principal actions. Understanding the basics of these cause-and-effect relationships will allow the reader to appreciate more fully the phenomena of ginger's therapeutic benefits.

From Action to Effect

Ginger's enzyme principal action is a good example of an action-to-effect dynamic.[12]

One of the previously described constituents that participates in ginger's principal enzyme action is called zingibain. Since one gram of zingibain can actually tenderize as much as twenty pounds of meat, improved digestion would be the most obvious impact or observed effect. Besides improving digestion, ginger's principal enzyme action also undoubtedly contributes to its combination of antibacterial,[13] anthelmintic[14] and anti-inflammatory[15] observed effects.

Numerous studies have shown that enzymes like zingibain can enhance the effectiveness of other antibacterial elements such as antibiotics[16] by as much as 50 percent.[17] To help eliminate parasites, an enzyme like zingibain can also aid the immune system by potentially digesting the parasite and its eggs.[18] Lastly, proteolytic enzymes are often associated with significant anti-inflammatory activity.[19]

From Effect Back to Action

One of ginger's most pronounced observed effects is its ability to counter inflammation. It also provides an excellent example of an observed effect with a profound interplay of *root* principal actions. At least three principal actions including 1) antioxidant, 2) enzyme and 3) eicosanoid balance are at work. As a powerful antioxidant,♦ with more than twelve constituents superior to vitamin E,[20] ginger helps neutralize free radicals which are widely recognized as participating or

---

♦ Ginger's antioxidant action is thought to result from a number of constituents including zingerone.

being responsible for the inflammatory process (*see chart 7: The Antioxidant Properties of Ginger*). Ginger's enzyme action combines, in an intricate interplay mirroring a Rube Goldberg♦ invention, with at least four other synergists to in turn affect another principal action involving critically important inflammation-related elements called eicosanoids.[21]

From just these two examples it should be clear that it would be a Herculean task to connect all of a plant's individual elements with principal actions and then in turn with clinically observed effects. Although it is a valuable exercise, it is not attempted here. With this reasoning in mind, please note *figure 5, The Principal Actions of Ginger*, and *figure 6, Ginger's Demonstrated Effects*.

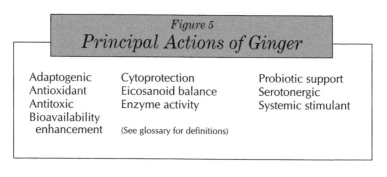

Figure 5
Principal Actions of Ginger

Adaptogenic	Cytoprotection	Probiotic support
Antioxidant	Eicosanoid balance	Serotonergic
Antitoxic	Enzyme activity	Systemic stimulant
Bioavailability		
enhancement	(See glossary for definitions)	

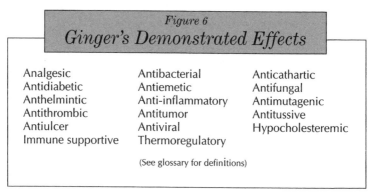

Figure 6
Ginger's Demonstrated Effects

Analgesic	Antibacterial	Anticathartic
Antidiabetic	Antiemetic	Antifungal
Anthelmintic	Anti-inflammatory	Antimutagenic
Antithrombic	Antitumor	Antitussive
Antiulcer	Antiviral	Hypocholesteremic
Immune supportive	Thermoregulatory	

(See glossary for definitions)

♦ Rube Goldberg was the American sculptor who created extremely complex diagrams of contraptions designed to effect relatively simple results.

The $70 Billion Challenge

❧NOTE❧
One of the body's most important chemical reactions
involves compounds called eicosanoids. When these
elements derived from dietary fat are out of balance,
many different disease conditions can evolve. Two of
the most threatening are heightened inflammation
and a more viscous or clot-prone blood. To a person
who is susceptible to arthritis or heart disease, the
results of this imbalance could be devastating. Drug
companies have spent many billions of dollars unsuc-
cessfully attempting to manipulate this balance safely
and effectively.

Introduction

There is little doubt that one key to understanding not only
the benefits of ginger but also the dynamics of our overall
health is to appreciate compounds known as eicosanoids.
Eicosanoids are those physiologically active compounds pos-
sessing a hormonal or regulatory-type nature, which are
enzymatically produced from dietary fat and principally from
an essential fatty acid called arachidonic acid. Eicosanoids
are broken down by structure and their catalyst enzymes
into three major groups called prostaglandins, thromboxanes
and leukotrienes (*see chart 1: The Eicosanoid Cascade*).
These three principal groups of eicosanoids interact with one
another in virtually every organ system of the body. As
tempting as it is to classify one eicosanoid as *positive* and
another as *negative*, the reality is that the ratio or proportion
with the others is probably most critical.♦ For health to be
preserved, there is little doubt that a balance of these compounds must be maintained. Even from the very beginning of

---

♦ Even the leukotrienes, which are usually blamed for chronic inflammatory conditions such
as asthma, rheumatoid arthritis, psoriasis and inflammatory bowel disease,[22] clearly play a
role in the destruction of harmful materials and contribute to tissue repair and healing.

life, eicosanoids are locked in an interplay with dramatic potential (*see chart 2, The Basic Functions of Eicosanoids, and chart 3, The Impact of One Eicosanoid and Enzyme*).✦

Fantastic Failure

The pharmaceutical industry has recognized that eicosanoid manipulation is a key to the normal functioning of many body systems, particularly the inflammatory process and cardiovascular system. Because of this, they have attempted to modulate or inhibit eicosanoid enzymes. To date, at least two hundred drugs[23] have been specifically designed to manipulate eicosanoids or relieve the inflammatory process at a current marketing and development cost as high as *$70 billion*.

Unfortunately, the drug companies have encountered serious problems when trying to manipulate these enzymes.[24] When the enzyme thromboxane synthetase is inhibited to minimize thromboxanes, other contracting and aggregating prostaglandin-type substances called prostaglandin endoperoxides replace the thromboxanes.[25] To make matters worse, the thromboxane synthetase inhibitors are also known to hamper normal removal of calcium from cells.[26] When the alternative cyclooxygenase enzyme is checked to minimize both prostaglandins and thromboxanes, there are also serious side effects. Well-known cyclooxygenase inhibitors are drugs referred to as nonsteroidal anti-inflammatory drugs (NSAIDs), which include aspirin, ibuprofen and indomethacin.⊐ NSAIDs reduce all prostaglandins, including the

---

✦ PGI_2 (also called prostacyclin) and TXA_2 are important regulators of the fetal blood supply. PGI_2 dilates and makes the blood less sticky, while TXA_2 constricts and causes blood to aggregate or clot. In reproductive tissues in a normal pregnancy, PGI_2, which is widely accepted as being a most important prostaglandin, dominates TXA_2. During complications with pregnancy like preeclampsia and multiple abortions, this ratio shifts and TXA_2 increases while PGI_2decreases. It is not surprising then that the insidious habit of cigarette smoking, which also increases the TXA_2 to PGI_2 ratio, is likewise associated with increased birth defects.[27]

⊐ It is ironic that we take NSAIDs drugs (i.e., aspirin and acetaminophen) during a cold, when research demonstrates that these drugs might actually be lengthening the duration of a cold's uncomfortable symptoms.[28] Of even greater concern is regular intake of NSAIDs such as aspirin which are associated with an alarming ten-fold increase in women and four-to - eight-fold increase in men of renal pelvic cancer.[29] Although the mechanism for this carcinogenic effect is not entirely clear, it appears that aspirin inhibits the clearance of a urine component called creatinine.

good mucus-protective PGI_2. Without PGI_2 there will be a deterioration of the mucus lining and a real danger of potentially fatal ulcers, which have become almost synonymous with the intake of NSAIDs.[30] Lipoxygenase inhibitors, as well as virtually all other anti-inflammatory protocols, have also either not met expectation or been rejected for numerous reasons. While lipoxygenase inhibitors failed to make it to human trials due to toxicity,[31] other classes of anti-inflammatory drugs like immunosuppressants and corticosteroids have left a legacy of adverse side effects including hypertension, brittle bones and thin skin.[32] While these side effects are a serious problem, a more dangerous potential lies in how these drugs affect the immune system. Eicosanoids play a key role in immunity, and their chemical inhibition could dramatically weaken normal immune function.[33]

A Key to the Vault

❧NOTE❧

While billions of dollars are being invested in modern pharmaceutical eicosanoid manipulation, poor results and toxicity have created a great potential for natural alternatives. Although a recent focus on essential fatty acid manipulation has been promising, a natural enzymatic approach has been relatively ignored. Remarkably, we have a diamond in our spice cabinet and virtually no one knows it. More than twelve studies have shown that ginger, like some of our most powerful pharmaceuticals, can positively affect this most critical of physiological reactions.

While chemical drug manipulation of eicosanoids has met with accumulating obstacles, research exploring safer and ultimately more effective alternatives in the field of nutritional science has intensified. Most of the research has focused on the dietary fat-EFA-eicosanoid connections by incorporating vegetable and marine source oils like that from cod, evening primrose, and flaxseed into the diet. The fundamental theory is that if the substrate arachidonic acid can be replaced or reduced by other essential fatty acids (dietary fat management), then there will be less inflammatory-type eicosanoids produced (*see chart 1: The Eicosanoid Cascade*). Although the clinical research is promising,[34] the results are still not conclusive.[35]

A brief study of the eicosanoid cascade strongly suggests that there is another approach that might be superior or, at least, complementary to dietary fat management. This method would be to affect the cascade closer to the source or at the enzymes themselves, essentially taking the same angle as the drug companies, albeit with natural agents. Some effort has been made in this direction with botanicals like meadowsweet herb and white willow bark, which might inhibit the cyclooxygenase and lipoxygenase enzymes; but the research is still lacking confirmation and safety of universal application.

The most remarkable and probably important principal action of ginger is that it is a profound and safe modulator or balancer of the vital eicosanoid cascade. Through its inhibition of at least two eicosanoid enzymes, 5-lipoxygenase and cyclooxygenase, ginger has been shown in at least twelve studies to correct or balance eicosanoid ratios. Ginger inhibits excesses of thromboxanes and leukotrienes such as TXA_2 and LTB_4 while allowing vital prostaglandins like PGI_2 to remain dominant or be minimally affected.[36] Estimates range from a 60 percent inhibition of thromboxanes to a 56 percent inhibition in specific inflammatory-type prostaglandins[37] (*see chart 4, Ginger's Effect on Specific Eicosanoids*). Ginger also reduced the substitute inflammatory compounds called prostaglandin endoperoxides, which plague modern chemical pharmaceutical thromboxane synthetase inhibitors.[38] One study showed that as many as four constituents of ginger were actually more potent inhibitors of prostaglandins than indomethacin, "which is known as one of the strongest (chemical) eicosanoid inhibitors."[39] Considering the fact that indomethacin has annual sales approaching $100 million, our common spice begins to show its competitive potential. Most remarkably, ginger achieves its no-side-effect[40] eicosanoid impact with a startling array of physiological benefits ranging from immune enhancement to gastroprotection. *This single statement is one of the most impressive in this book.* Where $70 billion worth of modern pharmaceuticals have essentially failed safely and effectively to balance eicosanoids, a common spice proves to possess a phenomenal and superior potential.

4

A HEALER FOR 5,000 YEARS

꙰꙰꙰꙰

The Rise and Fall of Ginger

Ginger is perhaps the best and most *sattvic*
[life-supporting] of the spices. It was called *vishwabhesaj*,
the universal medicine.

DR. VASANT LAD[1]

❧NOTE❧

Thousands of years of reverence are understandable
when one considers how ginger has helped humanity.
From Confucius and Hippocrates to the observations
of 25,000 Eclectic physicians of the early twentieth
century, the historically revered values of ginger are
simply fantastic. From spiritual beverage to aphrodisiac to remedy extraordinaire, ginger represents a
healing heritage that is virtually unmatched in the history of medicine. This section differs from the next in
that the reports are neither recorded in a published
study nor the subject of modern methods of scientific
investigation.

Introduction

Of all spices or herbs, the medical history of ginger is one of the richest in detail and personality. From the earliest written records to modern times, the following are the cumulative observations or records of millions of people through thousands of years. The way ginger has been used historically is virtually endless. In an attempt to put this enormous record into perspective, this chapter highlights a few of the most remarkable instances and themes throughout the body of ginger literature *(see figure 7)*.

For Spiritual Upliftment

The earliest written archives of the medicinal use of ginger come from the traditional Chinese and Ayurvedic Indian systems. Both systems clearly viewed ginger as a healing gift from God. According to one of the most ancient Chinese pharmacopoeias, long-term usage of fresh ginger would put a person in contact with the spiritual effulgences.[2] In ancient India, ginger was given the name *vishwabhesaj*, the universal medicine, and was viewed as an essential element in a majority of formulations.[3] Centuries later, the sacred writings of the Koran declared ginger a beverage of the holiest heavenly spirits. Considering how ginger has helped humanity, these thousands of years of spiritual reverence are understandable.

For Digestive Comfort and Strength

Virtually every cultural ethnomedical record, from the writings of Confucius to current times, has recognized and applauded the digestive benefits of consuming ginger. One would be hard-pressed to find a single culture that has been touched by ginger that has not reported its profound digestive stimulant or tonic, soothing and protective benefits. As early as 500 B.C. Confucius wrote that he was never without ginger when he ate. Dioscorides, referred to as the surgeon general for emperors Claudius and Nero, wrote in the famous *De Materia Medica* in 77 A.D. that ginger "warms and softens the stomach."[4] In one of the best reviews of the history of ginger's applications, Bruce Cost writes that ginger was regarded as the "Alka-Seltzer of the Roman Empire."[5]

Jumping millennia into the archives of U.S. history, the name *ginger* was virtually synonymous with digestive benefit. Ginger rations were part of the Revolutionary War soldier's diet. As a condiment jam, ginger graced dinner tables in New England to help prevent after-meal belching and flatulence. As herbal medicine reached its peak of acceptance in the U.S. in the early twentieth century, ginger was regarded as an herb of choice for digestive support (*see figure 8*).

> It is of an heating and digesting qualitie, and is
> profitable for the stomacke.
>
> JOHN GERARD, 1597[6]

Loving with Ginger

An interesting and consistent theme running throughout the historical literature is ginger's reputed value as an aphrodisiac. From the earliest recorded herbal formulations of India and China to its more modern applications in the Middle East and Cuba, ginger's millennia-long reputation as an aphrodisiac is impressive. The list of references on ginger's sexual tonic properties include endorsements by the Greek Dioscorides; a citation in Arabia's *A Thousand and One Nights*; John Gerard's◆ prescriptive herbal; and Italy's famed University of Salerno which influenced the direction of European health care for approximately one thousand years. This pioneering medical school prescribed that a rule for happy life in old age was to "eat ginger, and you will love and be loved as in your youth."[7] This sentiment was reiterated in *The Perfumed Garden*, a fourteenth-century sex manual which stated that "a man

---

◆ The famous English herbalist and author of *The Herball,* who wrote of ginger as "provoking venerie."[8]

who prepared himself for love with ginger and honey would give such pleasure to the woman that she would wish the act to continue forever."

Ginger's perceived property as an aphrodisiac helped determine its degree of cultivation and cultural popularity. It was ginger's sexual-tonic properties that were reportedly instrumental in encouraging the Portuguese to cultivate the spice in West Africa. Treating people much like cattle, these colonialists would feed the men in slave camps ginger with the goal of increasing populations and profits. Interestingly, one of the principal reasons cited for the decline of ginger's widespread use in the late seventeenth century was the transition from "the lusty Elizabethans giving way to the Puritans and later the Victorians . . . where the unabashed use of aphrodisiacs became frowned upon." [9]

Ginger's reputation as an aphrodisiac is undoubtedly connected to its widespread use as a systemic tonic.♦ In China, ginger has long been regarded as an agent to stimulate appetite, improve circulation and balance hormonal flow. In neighboring Tibet, ginger earned regard for strengthening the vital energies of the debilitated and lethargic.[10] In the Middle East, historians of ancient cultures like Persia wrote that ginger was valued for its properties of clearing the brain. It can be easily argued that all of these observed benefits would be prerequisites or synergists to a healthy sexual appetite.

Keeping the Peace

The last major category in the groupings of ginger's historic benefits can be termed infirmity relief. Around the world, ginger has been, either alone or in combination, the treatment of choice for virtually every type of pain or bodily discomfort. One of the greatest testimonials to ginger is that it still remains a component of more

---

♦ The word *tonic* is foreign to the current U.S. medical pharmacopoeia, where today the closest relative or last remnant is probably a cup of caffeine-rich coffee. Historically, and in virtually every other culture, myriad herbs were employed for their systemically strengthening effects.

than 50 percent of all traditional herbal remedies.[11] The Japanese soothed sore throats and spinal and joint pains, the Filipinos relieved headaches,[12] the Chinese countered toothache and the symptoms of a cold, flu and hangover, and the early-twentieth-century U.S. Eclectic physicians prescribed ginger for painful menstruation and as a remedy for breaking up colds.[13]

One of the most thought-provoking applications of ginger was that of fifth-century Chinese sailors. Approximately 1,200 years before the British surgeon Dr. James Lind discovered that a lime could prevent scurvy, the Chinese used ginger's vitamin C nutritive values for scurvy protection on long voyages.♦

The Fall of Ginger

What has become of ginger as a therapeutic entity? Why is it a mere shadow of its past?

The change in the seventeenth century's cultural outlook on aphrodisiacs is a factor. Far more significant, though, is the combination of the availability of fresh food and the recent era of miracle drugs.[14]

Before the modern era of sanitary food storage and fresh-food availability, spices played a critical role in food preservation and presentation.◻ Spices like ginger could both retard spoilage and disguise tastes. With fresh food becoming readily available, our once-glorious spices soon became regarded as an almost undesirable symbol, a mere accouterment to hide real flavors — or worse, a mark of underlying spoilage. Although this perception is no longer prevalent and the culinary value of spices is again enjoying recognition, their basic food-preservative or antioxidant values are still relatively ignored in favor of potentially toxic chemicals.

♦ As is so often the case, close mindedness blots the history of medicine. Not only was a scurvy remedy well known in European medicine at least one hundred years earlier [15] but James Lind and his simple prescription for scurvy were scorned for forty-eight years (until a year after his death). It is sobering to think of how many lives were needlessly lost because of this ignorance.[16]

◻ Recent studies at the University of California, Davis, demonstrated that when ginger was added to meat, the samples lasted three times longer.[17] Ginger's potent antioxidant properties were noted for this effect. Antibacterial and antifungal properties are also undoubtedly related to these food-preservative properties.

The most serious challenge to ginger and thousands of years of traditional medicine has been the modern era of miracle drugs, or magic bullets, and their concomitant regulatory and profit-motivated supporting institutions. With the discovery of drugs like antibiotics and corticosteroids, the industrialized world began what can only be described as an infatuation with the chemist's lab. Within as little as forty years, eons of traditional healing knowledge were virtually discarded in favor of isolated and synthesized chemical compounds. With worldwide medical traditions facing extinction, the last decade has seen a reawakening of interest in traditional remedies. Devastating side effects and poor results associated with many modern drugs and medical treatments are undoubtedly at the root of this resurgence. Whether this positive change will take hold, however, is yet to be determined (see chapter 8, "Freedom and Health at the Crossroads").

In Defense of History

Although many historic claims for ginger are not yet backed by double-blind placebo-controlled studies, this should not diminish the profound value of empirical observation. If a remedy is used for hundreds or even thousands of years for a particular purpose, it is highly doubtful that its popularity could be sustained if it were a placebo effect alone. Why would parents throughout history give their feverish children ginger if it didn't work? From the Admiralty Islands to Yemen, the list and longevity of traditionally tested treatments using ginger are truly monumental.

If a therapeutic application is used for the same purpose in completely different regions of the world, this clearly suggests there is authenticity to the usage. As an example, ginger has been used as a treatment for arthritis from Brazil to the Sudan to Papua-New Guinea, as an emmenagogue (to promote menstruation) from Venezuela to Vietnam, and as an aphrodisiac from Cuba to Yemen.

Lastly, it is undeniable that common sense plays a crucial part in the scientific method. Well-designed studies support or confirm many of the historic claims for ginger, and some of them are virtually irrefutable. Just as studies are unnecessary to substantiate the stimulant action of coffee or the laxative effect of prunes, many of ginger's values, such as its digestive benefits, are unequivocal.

Figure 7
Worldwide Appreciation for Ginger

Admiralty Islands:
contraceptive [18] (v)

Brazil:
bronchitis [19] (p)
rheumatism (p)

China:
digestive tonic [20]
emmenagogue [21] (ft)
thermoregulatory [22]

Cuba:
aphrodisiac [23] (ft)
emmenagogue (ft)
systemic stimulant (ft)

England:
morning sickness [24] (ft)

Fiji:
asthma [25] (j)
colds (j)
coughs (j)
earache (j)
stomachache (j)

India:
carminative [26]
colic
cough [20]
diabetes [27]
dietary vegetable [28] (v)
digestive stimulant [26]
childbirth [29] (j)
emmenagogue [30] (ft)
fever [20]
filariasis [31] (ft)
gingivitis [32] (j)
headache [26] (p)
nerve disorders [33]
rheumatism [20]
sore throat [29] (v)
stomach pain [26] (j)
tuberculosis [29] (v)

Japan:
hair growth [34] (p)

Indonesia:
colic [35] (j)
rheumatism (p)
snakebite (p)

Malaysia:
tonic after birth [36] (ft)

Mauritius:
emmenagogue [37] (dt)

Mexico:
digestive tonic [38] (ft)

Nigeria:
antimicrobial [39]
schistosomiasis [40] (dt)
wound healing [39]

Papua-New Guinea:
aching limbs [41] (p)
colds [42] (j)
coughs (j)
digestive healer [41] (ft)
digestive tonic [43] (dt)
fever [41] (ft)
malaria (j)
migraine [43] (p)
pneumonia [41] (ft)
poisonous stings [43] (p)

Continued on next page

Ginger has benefited humankind since the beginning of recorded history. With little difficulty, a book could be written covering all the different ways ginger has been used successfully throughout the ages. The above describes in one to two words a few of the cross-cultural usages as detailed in approximately fifty books or articles. The listing here is not meant to be all-inclusive and does not include any of the vast number of references for ginger in combination with other herbs.

Figure 7 — Continued

Papua-New Guinea (cont.)
rheumatism [41] (ns)
stomach worms [42] (v)
toothache [44] (ft)
topical ulcers [41] (p)
tuberculosis (ft)
vomiting [43] (j)

Peru:
carminative [45] (dt)
contraceptive [46] (dt)

Philippines:
childbirth pain [47] (dt)

Saudi Arabia:
anesthetic [48] (dt)
antiemetic [49] (dt)
antiseptic [48] (dt)
astringent (dt)
carminative [49] (dt)
digestive [50] (dt)
diuretic [48] (dt)

South Korea:
abortifacient [51] (dt)

Sudan:
colds [52] (dt)
pneumonia (dt)
rheumatism (dt)

Sumatra:
childbirth [36] (ft)

Tanganyika:
galactagogue [53] (ft)

Thailand:
antiemetic [54] (dt)
anticolic (dt)
carminative [55] (dt/ft)
cardiotonic [56] (dt)
diarrhea [57] (ft)
digestive [58] (dt)
emmenagogue [59] (ft)
fever [57] (ft)
headache [60] (p)

hypnotic [56] (dt)
postnatal [61] (dt)
tonic [62] (dt)

USA:
alcoholic gastritis [63]
antinausea
antipyretic
carminative [64] (dt)
cold remedy [65]
diaphoretic
digestive pain [12]
emmenagogue [66]
migraine

Venezuela:
emmenagogue [67] (ft)

Vietnam:
emmenagogue [68] (ft)

Yemen:
aphrodisiac [69]
stimulant (ft)

In this figure, ginger preparations for each application are indicated as: dt = dried tea; ft = fresh tea; j = juice; p = poultice; v = vegetable; ns = not stated in reference. First reference number includes all listings that follow until the next citation.

Figure 8
Quotations from the Eclectics

"When chewed it occasions an increased flow of saliva, and when swallowed it acts as a stimulating tonic, stomachic, and carminative, increasing the secretion of gastric juice, exalting the excitability of the alimentary muscular system, and dispelling gases accumulated in the stomach and bowels. . . . It is eminently useful in habitual flatulency, atonic dyspepsia, hysteria and enfeebled and relaxed habits, especially of old and gouty individuals; and is excellent to relieve nausea, pains and cramps of the stomach and bowels . . . especially when those conditions are due to colds. . . . ginger in the form of 'ginger tea' is popular and efficient as a remedy for breaking up colds, and in relieving the pangs of disordered menstruation."
Harvey Wickes Felter, M.D., and John Uri Lloyd, Phr.M., Ph.D.[70]

"The hot decoction of ginger tea is an excellent diaphoretic for breaking up incipient colds. It stimulates the circulation and the warmth it imparts to the body corrects the surface chilliness associated with colds....It stimulates the flow of the digestive juices and the warmth it imparts to the stomach is gratifying."
A. W. Kuts-Cheraux, N.D.[71]

"It is a profound and immediate stimulant, an active diaphoretic, an anodyne in gastric and intestinal pain, and a sedative to an irritated and overwrought system when there is extreme exhaustion."
Finley Ellingwood, M.D., and John Uri Lloyd, Ph.M., Ph.D., LL.D.[72]

The acceptance of ginger's healing properties reached its peak in the United States with references in multiple editions of Ellingwood's great tome Materia Medica Therapeutics and Pharmacognosy. *Finley Ellingwood, M.D., relied upon the observations of approximately 25,000 physicians, called Eclectics, to bring this work to completion. The quotes suggest a profound appreciation for ginger. While emphasis is placed on the digestive properties, some of ginger's sustained effects as an anti-inflammatory, systemic regulator and circulatory tonic were clearly noted.*

5

REFERENCES FOR A WONDER DRUG

୧(ଡ଼)ଡ଼

Relief for 27 Million Painful Days

After the diagnosis of rheumatoid arthritis all patients were treated with nonsteroidal anti-inflammatory drugs (NSAIDs) and some of the patients in later stages with corticosteroids and/or with gold salts. All the above management treatments only provided temporary relief. . . . Patient 1, an Asian male of fifty years of age living in Canada, was diagnosed as having rheumatoid arthritis. This patient began consumption of ginger in the first month following diagnosis by taking about fifty grams of fresh ginger daily after light cooking along with vegetables and various meats. . . . Pain and inflammation subsided after 30 days of ginger consumption. After consuming fifty grams of ginger daily for three months the subject was completely free of pain, inflammation or swelling. He has continued to perform his job as auto mechanic without any relapses of arthritis for the last 10 years.

Dr. K. C. Srivastava,
Danish Researcher[1]

✤NOTE✤

Modern medicine has had little to offer in treating arthritis, the nation's primary crippler. Side effects have plagued these conventional medications, killing thousands each year, and it is a rare event when the patient is actually healed. In two clinical trials conducted in Denmark, ginger actually reversed many of the subjects' arthritic symptoms and did so without side effects. Researchers attributed these benefits, among other possibilities, to the balancing of critical body enzymes.

The modern scientific method is beginning to demonstrate that the range of diseases that ginger can positively affect as an anti-inflammatory agent is staggering. Probably the most popular example of an inflammatory process is arthritis, the nation's primary crippler.[♦][2] Although more than 100 different diseases are grouped together under the designation of arthritis,[3] the common thread among them is inflammation and pain. It is estimated that 80 percent of persons over the age of fifty suffer from osteoarthritis,[4] while rheumatoid arthritis, a chronic inflammatory disease that affects the entire body including the joints, afflicts as many as 7 million in the United States.[5] Besides the incalculable cost of pain, arthritis is estimated to result in the loss of 27 million workdays or $8.6 billion in the U.S. alone.[6]

In the past one hundred years, there is hardly a question that there has been little progress in the treatment of arthritis. This is made painfully clear in a span of writings from a famous nineteenth-century British physician, Sir William Osler, to a current professor emeritus of medicine at the University of California, San Fransisco, Dr. Wallace Epstein.

> When a patient with arthritis walks in the front door, I
> feel like leaving out the back door.
> SIR WILLIAM OSLER[2]

♦ Other well-documented examples of chronic conditions with inflammation or eicosanoid imbalance at the root are asthma[7] and migraine headaches.[8]

> No one really knows whether prednisone, gold injections, methotrexate, sulfasalazine or hydroxychloroquine alter the joint destruction and deformity associated with the disease (arthritis)... Physicians do so [prescribe these remedies] without solid evidence that they do more good than harm in the long run. Ten years after commencing treatment, virtually no rheumatoid arthritis patients still take these medications, either because they do not work, or because of side effects.
>
> DR. WALLACE EPSTEIN[9]

How might a common spice transform this dismal picture? In an effect similar to aspirin and other NSAIDs, ginger reduces inflammatory eicosanoids like PGE_2, TXA_2 and LTB_4[♦9] (*See chart 4, Ginger's Effect on Specific Eicosanoids*). Amazingly, unlike these drugs which are plagued with side effects and diminished effectiveness,[□] ginger is not only safe and effective but it possesses a wide range of added benefits. Two clinical trials in Denmark underline this and strongly suggest that ginger should be included in all arthritis treatment programs.[10] (*See chart 5, The Effects of Ginger and Aspirin Compared, and chart 6, Ginger, Arthritis and Pain Relief*).[°]

In the first trial performed in 1989, seven rheumatic patients consumed fresh or powdered ginger for a period of three months. All patients reported that ginger produced better relief of pain, swelling and stiffness than the administration of NSAIDs. Remarkably six of these seven patients had been continuously afflicted with some degree of pain, inflammation, swelling and morning stiffness even after five to ten years of conventional treatment.

In the second trial involving fifty-six patients (twenty-eight with rheumatoid arthritis, eighteen with osteoarthritis and ten with muscular discomfort), the author K. C. Srivastava concluded that "more than three-quarters experienced,

---

♦ Danish researcher Srivastava proposes that ginger counters swelling or edema by inhibiting prostaglandins dilators like E2 and counters pain by reducing prostaglandin-mediated nerve endings sensitization to bradykinins.[11]

□ Research suggests that the use of NSAIDs in the treatment of arthritis may actually accelerate joint destruction.[12]

° A recently published case history of a migraine sufferer who experienced relief from ginger comparable to the drug dihydroergotamine adds another reference to ginger's anti-inflammatory potential.[13]

to varying degrees, relief in pain and swelling. All the patients with muscular discomfort experienced relief in pain." Although both Danish studies mostly attributed the benefits to balancing of eicosanoids, it can be argued that many other principal actions of ginger are at play.◆

An important note is that during the 2.5-year study period, no side effects were reported. Considering that, among the elderly alone, conventional arthritis treatment annually results in 3,300 NSAIDs-induced ulcer deaths,[14] ginger's advantage could not be clearer.

> Ginger produced better relief of pain, swelling and stiffness than the administration of NSAIDs . . . Some of our (arthritis) patients have observed added benefits on taking ginger, and they include relief in cold sores . . . fewer colds, amelioration of stomach irritation and constipation.
> K. C. Srivastava[10]

Your Heart Wants Ginger, NOT Aspirin

❊NOTE❊

Why is an outpatient cardiology clinic in an Israeli hospital now recommending to all its patients that they take one-half teaspoon daily of powdered ginger?[15] The answer is that ginger inhibits the same blood-thickening enzyme as aspirin and it accomplishes its task without side effects. Amazingly, ginger also offers a host of additional circulatory system benefits rivaling those of any natural treatment and transcending the potential of many modern cardiovascular drugs.

More than one-half of all deaths occurring in the United States annually are caused by clogged arteries. Included in

---

◆ The most obvious is ginger's principal antioxidant action. By countering free radicals which in turn stimulate inflammatory eicosanoids, joint-protective elements like hyaluronic acid are indirectly preserved.[16]

the catastrophic results of clogged arteries are heart attacks, coronary and cerebral thromboses, very high blood pressure, angina pectoris, shock, strokes and heart failure.[17]

A major contributor to clogged arteries is an excess of platelet-generated thromboxanes. Excess thromboxanes increase blood viscosity and aggregation leading to potentially lethal clotting. Many physicians now recommend the daily intake of acetylsalicylic acid (aspirin) to check this aggregation phenomenon and reduce the number of potentially fatal circulatory system events.

Because of aspirin's inhibitory effect on thromboxanes and prostaglandins, some experts estimate that regular consumption could prevent as many as 600,000 heart attacks a year, including 200,000 heart attack deaths. Research also suggests that regular consumption of aspirin could prevent up to 25,000 stroke-related deaths and as many as 24,000 deaths from colo-rectal cancer.[18] These potential benefits, however, could very well be overshadowed by significant systemic side effects.♦

The first documented report of ginger's enormous potential as a premier heart medicine came unexpectedly from a group of Cornell Medical School researchers and was published in the *New England Journal of Medicine* in 1980. The discovery occurred when one of the researchers noticed that his blood did not respond to the usual aggregating agents. After a process of elimination, he suspected that a 15 percent ginger marmalade was responsible. After challenging his platelet-rich plasma with ginger extract he confirmed that it completely inhibited the potentially life-threatening process of platelet aggregation.[19]

Numerous studies from around the world have corroborated the observations of the Cornell researchers. K.C. Srivastava wrote that even the smallest amount of ginger extract could abolish aggregation,[20] while other studies

---

♦ A major end point for judging aspirin's true effectiveness is to measure total mortality. Not surprisingly, some of the largest studies have demonstrated that regular aspirin consumers actually suffer a higher mortality rate.[21] Considering the greater exposure of regular aspirin consumers to bleeding ulcers, joint destruction and a potentially compromised immune system, the increased mortality is understandable.

confirmed that ginger and at least four of its constituents clearly possessed an aspirin-like effect in inhibiting platelet aggregation.[22] A recent Indian study published fourteen years after the Cornell research further underlined ginger's antiaggregatory potential. The work discovered that a daily supplement of 5 grams of powdered ginger, taken for seven consecutive days, significantly counteracted the blood platelet aggregating properties of 100 grams of butter and a chemical aggregating agent.[23] Compared in other studies to natural products, such as garlic, that are recommended for their antiaggregatory properties, ginger was found to be superior.[24]

The proverbial icing on the cake, which places ginger among the most exclusive class of healing herbs, is its other synergistic cardiovascular features. Ginger offers a profound antioxidant principal action and observed effects which include strengthening of the cardiac muscle[25] and lowering of serum cholesterol.[26]

As previously discussed, ginger is a powerful antioxidant, more so than even vitamin E or the chemical antioxidants BHA and BHT. If, as ongoing studies on tens of thousands of people suggest, even a small amount of antioxidants could offer up to a 40 percent reduction in cardiovascular disease,[27] then we have discovered the most critical justification for regular ginger supplementation.◆

Two studies in India and one in Japan, over a period of fifteen years, have shown that as a cholesterol-lowering agent, ginger and at least one of its constituents possess significant effects. In laboratory animals, ginger or its constituents reduced artificially elevated glucose levels by 51 percent. The mechanism for this action is not entirely clear, but it appears that ginger actually decreases or interferes with cholesterol biosynthesis.◻

◆ A recent Finnish study, widely reported in the media, has raised questions over the effect of isolated antioxidants in the prevention of lung cancer. Unfortunately the public was not informed that the researchers used dosages as low as 1/40th of previous studies and that there are serious study flaws using the Finnish population as a test case.[28] Regardless, one prescription is still unanimous; eat a diet as rich as possible in antioxidants.

◻ One study could not duplicate the cholesterol-lowering effects of ginger.[29] Many factors such as type of extract or dosage could explain this discrepancy.

Last, the term *cardiotonic* is often used in herbal medicine to characterize a botanical that is specifically beneficial to the cardiovascular system. Fascinating research performed at Tsumara Research Institute for Pharmacology and other Japanese universities has placed a modern twist on this terminology by declaring ginger a positive inotropic agent to the heart. This term means that ginger positively increases the force or strength of heart muscle tissue with an effect that has been likened to digitalis. Again, this extraordinary benefit is without side effects.

Whether the Heat Is High or Low

❊NOTE❊

Question: Why has ginger throughout time been a valuable aid in alleviating the fever and chills of colds?

Answer: Ginger reduces fever for the same reason that aspirin does. It inhibits the activity of a fever-causing enzyme.

Ginger possesses profound thermoregulatory properties.[30] Like aspirin and other NSAIDs which inhibit enzymes like cyclooxygenase and the production of certain inflammatory eicosanoids, ginger can alleviate the severity of a fever. When fever was induced in laboratory rats, ginger's effect was comparable to aspirin, reducing the fever by 38 percent[9] (*see chart 5: The Effects of Ginger and Aspirin Compared*). Besides reducing fever, historical and modern research show that ginger is also capable of relieving chills caused by the common cold and warming the body.[31]

Ginger's thermoregulatory properties may also have significant implications for those affected by obesity. According to published research from Australia, ginger warrants further investigation to assess its potential as a dietary antiobesity agent.[32]

Ulcers: #1 Drug Faces Contender

✶NOTE✲

Ginger combines two effects beyond the scope of any modern drug. It can relieve inflammation while simultaneously protecting the digestive system from ulcers. A modern drug may accomplish one or the other but never both. Ginger possesses the potential for both of these therapeutic benefits without the invasive realm of negative side effects.

The Final Word on NSAIDs

A medical knowledge that works–no matter how scientific
its origins–is a treasure that cannot be ignored.
Dr. HIROSHI NAKAJIMA, DIRECTOR GENERAL,
WORLD HEALTH ORGANIZATION.[33]

Whatever superiority NSAIDs have in the strength of their anti-inflammatory or thermoregulatory effects, ginger compensates for it with an absence of side effects and alternative benefits. One of these marked advantages is ginger's ulcer-preventive properties.[34] At least six antiulcer constituents from ginger have been isolated and identified.[35] Unlike NSAIDs which can cause life-threatening ulcers by inhibiting mucosal-protective prostaglandins, ginger actually upholds the integrity of the digestive tract mucosa.[36] Even when laboratory animals are exposed to severe stress, ginger extract can inhibit these ulcers by as much as 97.5 percent.♦

♦ One study[37] showed that ginger inhibited stress-induced ulcers from 25 to 55 percent, but the dosage was significantly lower (@62 mg/kg) than the cited study where the dosage was 1,000 mg/kg. A human equivalent of this dosage would be approximately 60 grams, which would appear to be excessive.

In this Japanese research, it was observed that two of ginger's most active constituents, [6]-gingerol and zingiberene, were not as effective as the whole extract, inhibiting gastric lesions by 53 and 54 percent respectively. This reduced effect supports the contention that the whole plant is superior to individual constituents.

NSAIDs may relieve inflammation but they all too often act like dominos. Their treatment course invariably leads to gastric irritation and another medication, in this case antiulcer drugs. One of the many justifications for declaring ginger a wonder drug is that while it is a potent anti-inflammatory agent, it might actually protect against NSAIDs-induced ulcers.[38] Please note that protecting against these particular ulcers is no minor achievement as they are recognized as being not only very dangerous but often unresponsive to H2-receptor antagonists[39] (*see chart 9, The Ulcer-Protective Spectrum of Ginger*).

Ginger vs. H2s

For the 25 million American males and 12 million females who suffer from duodenal and gastric ulcers,[40] the daily consumption of ginger offers an attractive alternative to Zantac® (ranitidine), Pepcid® (famotidine) and Tagamet® (cimetidine).♦ These three drugs, which are collectively referred to as H2-receptor antagonists, are notably among the twenty top-selling drugs in the U.S. and account for more than $2.8 billion in sales annually[41] (*see chart 10, The Twenty Top-Selling Drugs for 1992*).

Ginger has distinct advantages over these H2-receptor antagonists.◻ Besides its observed effect against NSAIDs-induced ulcers and its lack of side effects, ginger has two other benefits in its favor: 1) more optimal maintenance of pepsin-pH parameters; and 2) synergistic components (*see the section "Beyond Ulcers," on page 41*).

To appreciate fully the decided advantage of ginger over H2-receptor antagonists, a look at how these two elements achieve their effect is necessary. Cimetidine is a good example of the H2s' method of action because it is specifically compared with ginger in the research.

♦ Zantac® is a registered trademark of Glaxo Inc., Pepcid® is a registered trademark of Merck and Co. and Tagamet® is a registered trademark of Smithkline Beecham.

◻ The advantage of ginger over H2s as a protective agent against ulcers would probably be even greater with the simple addition of licorice. Numerous studies on licorice and its constituents show a profound healing property once lesions have formed.[42]

What ginger and cimetidine have in common is: 1) they reduce the total volume of gastric juices;[42]♦ and 2) they possess ulcer-protective properties. By reducing total gastric volume, cimetidine and ginger clearly minimize the digestive tract's exposure to irritation. While in one study cimetidine showed greater activity against severe lesions, its potential for negative impact on the enzyme pepsin could easily offset this advantage▢ (see chart 8, Ginger's Effect on Digestive Function).

As if side effects and compromised digestion were not enough to make one skeptical of H2s, consumers of these drugs ultimately have to deal with a poor long-term prognosis and significant expense. According to a recent report in U.S. News & World Report, these drugs are some of our most unsuccessful and expensive to use.[43] The report confirms that up to 90 percent of the people on these drugs suffer high recurrence rates and consumption over a fifteen year period may cost in excess of $10,000. Considering the contrast between a dismal array of antiulcer drugs and a promising list of ginger studies, it is hoped that controlled human trials will soon be initiated.

> Whatever elements nature does not introduce in
> vegetables, the natural food of all animal life–directly of
> herbivorous, indirectly of carnivorous–are to be
> regarded with suspicion.
> OLIVER WENDELL HOLMES, 1861[44]

♦ Ginger's exact effects on digestive secretions are still not conclusive.[45] One interesting conclusion from the research is that different extraction mediums can dramatically affect ginger's actions. For example, an alcohol extract will significantly reduce pepsin concentration compared to a water extract, while the reverse is true for gastric HCL concentrations. The same is true for eliciting ginger's cholagogic effect. An acetone extract produced significant effect while a water extract had no effect.[46]

▢ Pepsin is essential to split dietary protein into smaller molecules. For it to be active, though, the medium must be acidic. If gastric pH rises, or becomes less acidic, pepsin's activity decreases. In laboratory rats, cimetidine caused a 92 percent increase in pH to 4.2, while with ginger, the levels remained constant with controls at pH 2.3.[50] Short- and long-term ramifications of this increased pH and less active pepsin, although seldom studied and as yet not verified, could potentially be quite significant. These include: compromised absorption of dietary protein, vitamin B_{12} and iron, and an increase in opportunistic infections of the digestive tract.[47]

How an Herbalist Spells Relief

❧NOTE❧

To call ginger a digestive herb is an understatement. In addition to protecting against ulcers, ginger possesses a remarkable capability of treating opposites or balancing the system. Ginger can protect while it stimulates, inhibit toxic bacteria while it promotes friendly species and be effective in treating conditions ranging from constipation and diarrhea to the debilitating experience of nausea.

Beyond Ulcers

From all parts of the world, virtually every ethnomedical text citing ginger has lauded its wide range of benefits to the digestive system. A review of the current scientific literature clearly supports these empirical observations. Modern research shows that ginger's therapeutic range completely overshadows the potential of antiulcer H2-receptor antagonists. Included in its vulnerary profile are enzyme-enhanced protein digestion,[48] digestive stimulation,[49] antidiarrheal activity,[50] probiotic support,[51] liver protection[52] and antiemetic[53] properties. Interestingly, known side effects of H2-receptor antagonists include diarrhea, nausea and hepatotoxicity,[54] problems that consumption of ginger can actually address.

The first two benefits mentioned above, enzyme action and digestive stimulation, are direct synergists to ginger's previously mentioned antiulcer benefits. Like the H2-receptor antagonists, ginger does reduce a potentially important gastric volume. To compensate for this effect, ginger's abundant enzymes promote protein digestion, while its stimulant actions increase bile secretion. According to a group of Japanese researchers, ginger will therefore facilitate absorption of fat and electrolytes. A side benefit of increased bile secretion will be the relief of constipation and excretion of small gallstones.[55]

Another aspect of ginger, which might have antiulcer synergy and counter such varying conditions as diarrhea and constipation, is its principal probiotic and antitoxic actions.[56] A new theory that is gaining widespread recognition proposes that bacteria called Helicobacter pylori play a material role in the development of peptic ulcers.[57] Although there are no specific studies on ginger and this particular bacterial species, ginger has been shown to possess significant activity against a wide range of gram-negative and gram-positive bacteria. These pathogenic species include Escherichia coli, Proteus vulgaris, Salmonella typhimurium, Staphylococcus aureus and Streptococcus viridans.[58] Interestingly, while ginger is clearly inhibitory to these pathogenic species, it actually appears to stimulate the growth of potentially beneficial Lactobacillus species, which have been found to be useful in the treatment of both diarrhea and constipation.[59] Such is the wisdom of nature (*see figure 9*).

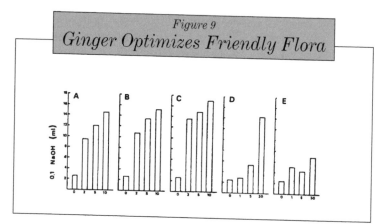

Figure 9
Ginger Optimizes Friendly Flora

A= pepper, B=cinnamon, C=ginger, D=garlic powder, E=fresh garlic extract
Of all tested spices, ginger most encourages the growth of a friendly flora species, Lactobacillus plantarum. Remarkably, ginger is simultaneously antimicrobial against toxic bacteria like E. coli.[60]

What Do Ocean Travel and Pregnancy Have in Common?

Of all ginger's effects, its antiemetic or antinausea property is probably the best known today. Thanks to the pioneering work of Daniel Mowrey, which demonstrated
ginger's superiority to dimenhydrinate,[61] it is becoming
increasingly common to see people taking ginger capsules
on long car trips or boat rides. Although this work has met
with recent controversy,[62] the body of research, including
both laboratory animal and human studies, strongly suggests that ginger is an effective aid to counter nausea and
vomiting. Whether the nausea results from chemotherapy,
ocean travel, pregnancy *(see the section "Safety First," on
page 87)* or gynecological surgery, ginger is clearly the
treatment of choice.

It is currently reported that up to 90 percent of all
patients receiving chemotherapy suffer from nausea and
vomiting. At the University of Alabama in 1987, researchers
reported that patients who received additional ginger
reported less severity and duration of nausea.[63] The Alabama work was supported by a Japanese study in 1989, where
researchers concluded that in laboratory animals, ginger
was the first natural medicine to be reported to antagonize
the profound emesis caused by a chemotherapeutic agent.[64]

When eighty Danish naval cadets, unaccustomed to
sailing in heavy seas, were studied to test the benefit of
ginger, researchers concluded that without side effects,
ginger reduced the tendency to vomiting and cold sweat-
ing significantly better than a placebo did.[65]

For the nausea of pregnancy, ginger has offered relief to
innumerable women. Technically referred to as hyperemesis gravidarum, nausea and vomiting can complicate up to
50 percent of normal pregnancies. A double-blind randomized crossover trial in England concluded that ginger
scored significantly greater results for relief of symptoms
than a placebo. When the women were asked their choices,
70.4 percent preferred ginger while only 29.6 percent had
no preference or selected the placebo treatment.[66]

Ginger has also been used successfully to treat the 30 percent incidence of serious nausea caused by major gynecological surgery, a condition for which there has been no real reduction in the last fifty years.[67] In sixty women who experienced this debilitating side effect, researchers found that there were significantly fewer recorded incidences of nausea with ginger than with the placebo and that ginger was comparable to the drug metoclopromide.[68] Three years later, a group of English researchers actually showed that ginger was superior to the drug metoclopromide (annual U.S. sales are approximately $23 million) in preventing the incidence of postoperative nausea and vomiting.♦ An important note is that unlike ginger which has only additional benefits, metoclopromide has a long list of side effects including mental depression and tardive dyskenesia.[69]

The conflicting works of Wood and Stewart[70] to those of Mowrey and Grontved[71] suggest that the effectiveness of ginger in treating motion sickness might be dependent upon a number of factors, the most important being the length of prior consumption. For optimal results, research indicates that dosing should begin at least three hours prior to the challenging event.[72]

A Pause on Nausea

The underlying mechanisms that can explain ginger's antiemetic properties are complex and controversial but important. Although ginger has been demonstrated to counteract nausea, its most pronounced effects are against vomiting.[73] Both nausea and vomiting can arise from many factors — the most common being the combination of food in the stomach and rapid motion or stress. Two obvious actions of ginger that might empty the stomach more quickly are its digestive enzyme and stimulant actions. Enzymes catalyze the stomach's protein digestion while

♦ The placebo, metoclopromide and ginger had respective incidence of nausea at 41, 27 and 21 percent.

stimulating pungent compounds enhance transport.[73]♦

While digestive stimulation and enzymes play a role in preventing nausea, the most interesting and probably important action attributed to ginger's antiemetic effects involves the metabolism of a well-known blood-platelet-derived storage product called 5-HT (5-hydroxytryptamine), or serotonin. It has been reported that ginger modulates or, more technically, acts as an antagonist at receptor sites of this amine (hereby referred to as 5-HT action),[74] explaining ginger's effectiveness in treating not only nausea[75] but a number of other digestive conditions ranging from constipation to diarrhea.⊐

Interestingly, ginger's 5-HT action has a broad range of added potential effects besides countering emesis including anti-inflammatory,[76] antiulcer,[77] antiaggregatory,[78] antiasthmatic,[79] blood pressure normalization[80] and preventing potentially fatal cerebral vasospasms.[81] Not surprisingly, the first three effects of this particular 5-HT action have already been demonstrated as benefits of ginger in the research.

Double Your Investment

❊NOTE❊

There is an old expression that you are what you eat. A more recent adaptation of this adage is that you are what you absorb. Ginger holds a millennia-old reputation as a carrier herb, an herb that enhances the absorption of other herbal elements. This feature is pertinent or vital to people taking dietary supplements or who have weak digestive systems. Studies suggest that daily consumption of ginger might enhance digestive absorption by as much as 200 percent.

♦ Ginger's antiemetic effect might very well be due to increased GI motility;[82] however, this effect is still unclear.[83] British researcher A. B. Lumb proposes in a letter in the journal *Anaesthesia* that motility-enhancement might impact the whole gastrointestinal tract as opposed to the gastric region via competition at 5-HT receptor sites.[84]

⊐ Recent animal studies strongly suggest that an interplay of gingerols and shogaols is at the center of ginger's antiemetic effects.[85]

Why has ginger been included in the majority of traditional remedies for thousands of years? The explanation given by traditional healers is that ginger acts as a carrier and improves the value of all other herbs in a combination. Not surprisingly, modern research offers a justification for this empirical herbal observation.[86]

Attempting to understand the ancient Ayurvedic formulation technique, which widely prescribed ginger and two other herbs, a group of Indian researchers studied one of these herbs and a constituent. The herb, long pepper and its constituent piperine, were examined for their effects on drug absorption. Long pepper and piperine improved absorption of two different drugs by 233 percent and more than 100 percent, respectively. Researchers concluded that the combination of long pepper, black pepper and ginger, traditionally called *trikatu*, was included in multiple formulations for its bioavailability-enhancing effect.

The researchers in the Indian study theorized a four-part mechanism for the effects of trikatu: 1) promoting absorption from the gastrointestinal tract; 2) protecting the drug from being metabolized/oxidized in the first passage through the liver after being absorbed; 3) a combination of these two mechanisms; and 4) causing increased production of bile.[87]

Considering that some of ginger's components appear to be in the blood for several days,[88] it is not farfetched to propose that ginger's bioavailability effect might be a sustained one. Since it is common knowledge that vitamins and minerals will have little value if they are not properly absorbed, a practical and more natural application of ginger's absorption-accelerating capabilities would be the inclusion of ginger in one's daily supplement program to enhance nutrient bioavailability.♦

> Ginger is generally combined with herbs going into the
> abdominal area, because it is a carrier. Ginger is an herb
> which accentuates so many herbs.
> DR. JOHN CHRISTOPHER[89]

♦ Interestingly, ginger is also recognized in the cosmetic industry as a transdermal drug accelerator.[90]

Next: Unthinkable Worms

❉NOTE❉

Although parasites are an unpleasant topic, it is
unfortunately one that needs to be broached. Considering that 25 million Americans are potentially
afflicted, a daily preventive and possible curative is
definitely needed. Studies show that ginger is remarkably effective against some of the world's most dangerous parasites and, unlike virtually all antiparasitic
medications, it is without negative side effects.

An important property of ginger that affects all systems,
particularly the digestive, is its anthelmintic or antiparasitic effect.[91] The ramifications of this effect are more important than most people suspect. Jane Brody, a science writer
for the *New York Times*, recently summarized the magnitude of this issue:[92]

> Worms may be unthinkable in this cleanliness-obsessed soci-
> ety, yet an estimated 25 million Americans, many of them
> young children and many from middle-class and affluent
> families, are often unknowing hosts to tiny intestinal worms.
>
> *JANE BRODY*[92]

Brody's concern is echoed by other reputable sources
which concur that most available figures on the prevalence of parasitic infections in the U.S. are underesti-
mates[93] and that over one billion people in the world are
hosts to various types of worms.[94]

Clinical findings on ginger reveal that it possesses a broad
range of anthelmintic effects including activity against some
of the world's most widespread and dangerous parasites *(see
figure 10)*. This strong activity has been demonstrated with
nematodes or roundworms including Anisakis, Ascaris and
Filaria and trematodes or flatworms in the Schistosoma
genus. Although most of this work is performed using in-vitro tests, the results are promising and deserve further study.

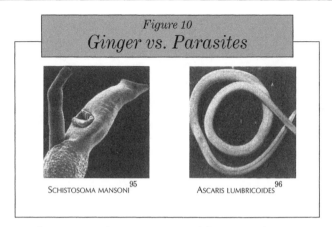

Figure 10

Ginger vs. Parasites

SCHISTOSOMA MANSONI[95]   ASCARIS LUMBRICOIDES[96]

Schistosoma and Ascaris are two of the principal parasites that collectively infect billions of people worldwide. Promising research indicates that ginger can inhibit or kill these dangerous parasites.

Reprinted with permission from **Medical Parasitology** by E. K. Markell, M. Voge, D.T. John, published by W.B. Saunders Co., Philadelphia, PA.,1986.

Ginger's anthelmintic effect is probably a consequence of a combination of principal actions including those that involve potent enzymes and pungent stimulants. A brief summary of the work follows:

- Anisakis, which is principally acquired through the consumption of sushi or raw fish, is an important parasitic infection in Japan and is increasing markedly in the US. Although the exact number of cases is unclear, no effective drug treatment exists to eliminate the worms which typically become embedded in the stomach or bowel wall. An in-vitro study demonstrated that an extract of ginger and two of its constituents caused more than 90 percent of the larvae to lose spontaneous movement within four hours and to be destroyed completely within sixteen hours.♦ Interestingly, pyrantel pamoate, an

---

♦ In this Japanese study, the combination of gingerol and shogaol constituents produced "synergistic effects." This is yet another example in favor of the contention that the whole plant is superior to any isolated active component.

antinematodal drug, had no lethal effect even at a relatively high concentration. It is therefore not surprising that ginger is traditionally eaten with sushi in Japan.

- Ascaris lumbricoides, which is lethal to approximately 20,000 people annually and affects an estimated one billion people worldwide, was effectively inhibited by ginger extract.[97]

- Filariae, which afflict at least 80 million people worldwide,[98] were effectively reduced in dogs by an extract of ginger by approximately 98 percent without any reported toxic effects.[99]

- Schistosoma, which is becoming increasingly prevalent in the U.S.,[100] is considered the second major parasitic disease in the world.[101] This infection is particularly insidious in that the parasite is capable of ingesting as many as 330,000 red blood cells per hour in a laboratory mouse.[102] Ginger "completely abolished" the infectivity in its early phases,[103] and in young children, ginger extract was found to significantly reduce the egg count in the urine indicating a systemic action.[104]

The Common Cold Meets Its Match

❧NOTE❧
The common cold has undoubtedly been a disagreeable aspect of the human condition since the beginning of recorded history. From the earliest written records to the conclusions of modern researchers, ginger has been recognized as an herb of choice for lessening the severity of a cold.

The pioneering work of the Danish researcher Srivastava established ginger as a powerful potential therapeutic tool for arthritis treatment. He also observed a side effect of ginger consumption that has been confirmed throughout the most ancient traditions of medicine. While subjects in Srivastava's studies reported a reduction in pain from arthritis, they also noticed that they contracted fewer or less severe colds or infections.[105] From the historic works of Ayurveda, to the writings of the Eclectic physicians of the early twentieth-century in the United States, these same observations have been made.

What are the principal actions behind ginger's cold-fighting properties? As with many of ginger's observed effects, a combination of principal actions including eicosanoid balance, cytoprotection and probiotic support is probably responsible. A case can also be made for its antitoxic principal action which encompasses ginger's distinct antibacterial,[106] antiviral,[107] and antifungal[108] observed effects.

Can one of the above principal actions be singled out as the most prominent? The best candidate would be eicosanoid balance with its anti-inflammatory and antipyretic benefits.[109] Just when one thinks, though, that a good choice has been made, another variable enters that might be equally important. For example, Japanese research in 1969 and 1984 determined that ginger possesses both a significant antihistaminic property[110] and an intense antitussive effect actually rivaling that of codeine.[111] Ultimately, as explanations mount for one of ginger's best-known effects, we can understand why the nineteenth-century Russian novelist Ivan Turgenev wrote, "However much you knock at nature's door, she will never answer you in comprehensible words."[112]

Getting at the Roots of Cancer

✻NOTE✻

It is widely believed that environmental exposure to toxins is responsible for as many as 80 percent of all cancers.[113] When tested against two accepted standards for toxicity, ginger significantly reduced their life-threatening potential. Ginger also possesses at least two other properties that could positively influence the course of a patient's cancer: 1) stimulation of immunity and 2) inhibition of platelet aggregation (preventing metastasis).

From Opposing Trp-P to Boosting Immunity

We are exposed to an endless variety of toxins in our air, water and food. The degree to which we are able to adapt to and detoxify these agents will to a major extent determine our quality of life and longevity. Two agents that are considered laboratory standards for creating toxicity are benzo(a)pyrene and pyrolysis products (burned by-products) of the amino acid tryptophan, commonly referred to as Trp-P. Trp-P is generally regarded as having a higher mutagenic or cancer-causing potential than benzo(a)pyrene.[114] Ginger, and a number of its constituents, showed remarkable effects[115] and were antimutagenic to both benzo(a)pyrene and (Trp-P).◆[115]

How the above detoxifying action might translate into a reduction in cancer is not clear. Ginger does appear to have some direct actions against certain forms of cancer which warrant further research.❏[115] For example, ginger extract extended the lifespan of laboratory animals induced with Dalton's lymphoma and Ehrlich ascites tumors by 11 percent.[116] While this is an intriguing result, the real promise that ginger holds in the field of cancer treatment revolves around two distinct effects, namely immune stimulation and inhibition of platelet aggregation.

A stronger immune system is obviously relevant to cancer because it can both help prevent carcinogenesis and it can extend the longevity of a cancer patient. Unlike any current eicosanoid-inhibiting anti-inflammatory drug,

---

◆ Further testaments to ginger's protective values are studies showing it can enhance survival to radiation[117] and decrease the potential toxicity of other herbs. When Rhizoma Pinelliae is immersed in ginger juice, its toxicity is significantly reduced.[118]

❏ Recent research also suggests that the eicosanoid-inhibiting properties of aspirin might be responsible for blocking a colon tumor's growth factors.[119]

Arabian researchers tested ginger for its effect on male rats. Not only was ginger absent of spermatotoxic effects, but it actually, according to the researchers, significantly increased the sperm motility and sperm contents[♦][131] *(see chart 11, Ginger and the Male Reproductive System).* Other factors, not directly associated with the sexual organs — namely, processes like improved systemic circulation and better digestion/nutrient bioavailability — provide additional bases for historically observed sexual tonic effects.

On a related note, ginger is used externally by traditional Oriental practitioners to affect a number of body functions including the reproductive system. A recent Chinese report on breech births underlines this potential. The study concluded that simply applying a ginger paste to a specific acupressure point in these pregnant women allowed a 77.4 percent correction rate, as opposed to the control group which had only a 51.6 percent correction rate.[132] Whatever the underlying reason for the correction of breech position "effect," it is clear that an external application of ginger may have surprising benefits.

♦ The Israeli researcher Joshua Backon has published a number of articles on ginger proposing that excess eicosanoids are partially responsible for impotence.[133] Dr. Backon also suggests that this same mechanism is responsible for menstrual cramping and discomfort.[134]

6
CHARTING GINGER'S ACCOMPLISHMENTS

❧❦❧

___❧NOTE❧___

This chapter includes eleven charts preceded by their explanations. These graphic displays emphasize the actions and benefits of ginger in various contexts.

Chart 1: The Eicosanoid Cascade

The three principal end products of the eicosanoid cascade are the leukotrienes, thromboxanes and prostaglandins. Prostaglandin endoperoxides act as intermediaries to thromboxanes and prostaglandins. The first observation about the existence of what are now known as prostaglandins (PG) was made in 1930 by North American scientists who showed that fresh human semen possessed biological activity. Now identifiable in virtually all body tissues, prostaglandins constitute a minimum of thirty different compounds. As can be seen from the chart, the production of prostaglandins is principally dependent upon the cyclooxygenase enzyme. Thromboxanes (TX), discovered approximately forty years later, are created from prostaglandin endoperoxides mainly by blood platelets. The enzymes cyclooxygenase and thromboxane synthetase are the key determinants in the production of thromboxanes. Leukotrienes (LT), first isolated from white blood cells and often blamed for a host of inflammatory conditions, are principally dependent upon the 5-lipoxygenase enzyme.♦

A dual approach to the eicosanoid cascade, which includes both dietary fat management (reduction of arachidonic acid) and inhibition of eicosanoid enzymes, is clearly essential for optimal health. Through ginger's actions at the enzyme level of the eicosanoid cascade, inhibiting both COX and 5-LO, the result is a reduction or balancing of thromboxanes, leukotrienes and prostaglandins.

Chart 2: The Basic Functions of Eicosanoids

Eicosanoids play a diverse and complicated role in virtually every physiological function. One prostaglandin can mediate inflammation while another protects the mucus lining. It is therefore clear why we experience such serious side effects when all eicosanoids are inhibited.

♦ Other enzymes involved in eicosanoid synthesis are: E2 isomerase, I2 synthase, 12-lipoxygenase and cytochrome P-450. The number at the end of the eicosanoid (i.e., I2) signifies the number of double bonds in the side chain.

Chart 3: The Impact of One Eicosanoid and Enzyme

Just one eicosanoid and enzyme can have a profound influence on human physiology. The Israeli researcher Joshua Backon[1] describes a sampling of these effects arising from modulation of the prostaglandin PGI_2 and the enzyme thromboxane synthetase. Most remarkably, unlike NSAIDs, which interfere with PGI_2, ginger allows this eicosanoid to maintain its dominance.

Despite the fact that it is currently not clear whether ginger directly inhibits (TS), it will inevitably act as if it has. Ginger inhibits COX, which in turn reduces prostaglandins. Since prostaglandin endoperoxides are the starting material for thromboxanes, a lessening in prostaglandin endoperoxides will inevitably result in a reduction of thromboxanes. It is hard to believe that everything from anxiety to sudden death can be attributed to an excess of thromboxanes.◆

Chart 4: Ginger's Effect on Specific Eicosanoids

Whether in a test tube (in vitro) or in the blood of human subjects (ex vivo), there is little doubt that ginger reduces the levels of specific eicosanoids. Estimates range from a 60 percent inhibition of thromboxanes to a 56 percent inhibition in specific inflammatory-type prostaglandins.

References: In Vitro and On Three Prostaglandins[2] Ex Vivo[3]

Chart 5: The Effects of Ginger and Aspirin Compared

Two observed effects of reduced levels of eicosanoids would be a pronounced lessening in inflammation and fever. As expected, ginger is associated with both effects and is comparable to NSAIDs like aspirin. This study does not illustrate what potentially higher doses of ginger might offer. Clearly, the value and toxicity of aspirin peak much earlier.

Reference: Anti-inflammatory Effect and Antipyretic Effect[4]

◆ Please note that another enzyme, thromboxane synthetase, is responsible for converting prostaglandin endoperoxides into thromboxanes. Whether ginger also modulates this enzyme is not clear at this time.

The Eicosanoid Cascade

Dietary Fat (Essential Fatty Acids) to:

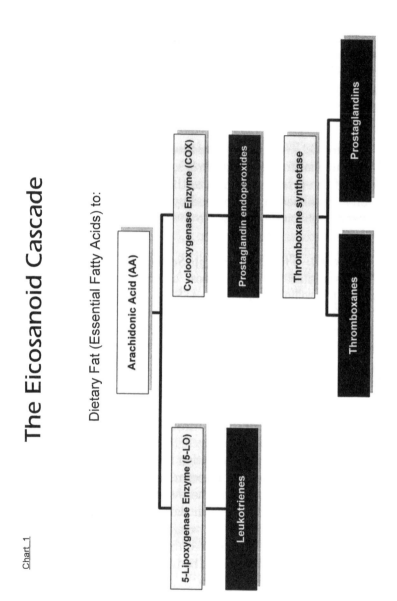

Chart 1

Chart 2

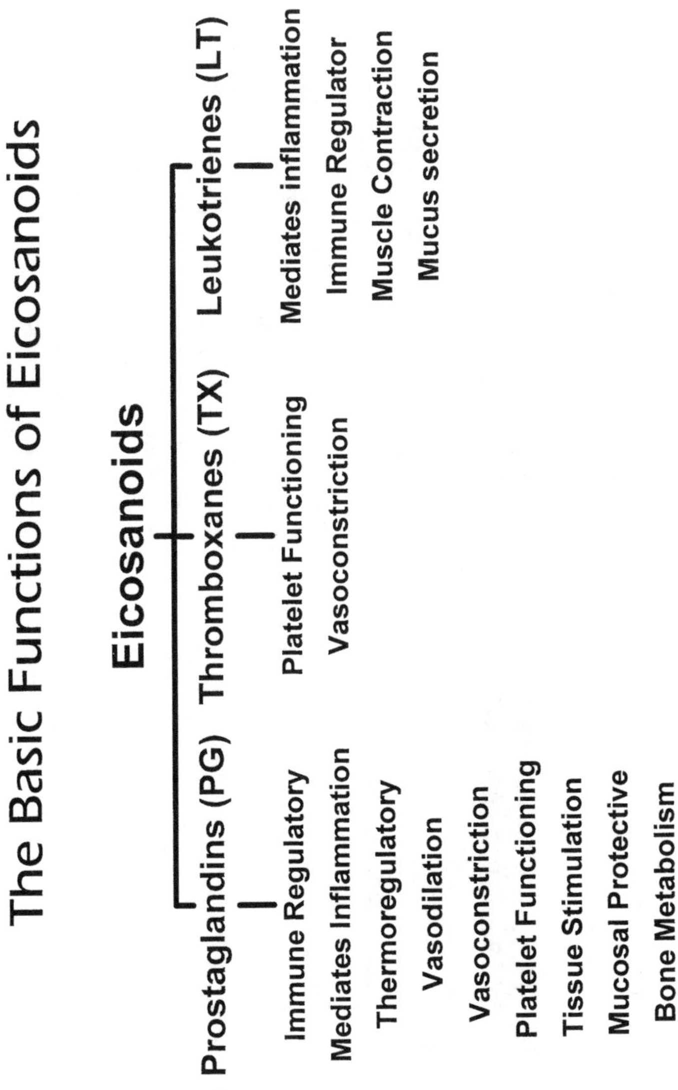

The Basic Functions of Eicosanoids

Eicosanoids

Prostaglandins (PG)

Immune Regulatory

Mediates Inflammation

Thermoregulatory

Vasodilation

Vasoconstriction

Platelet Functioning

Tissue Stimulation

Mucosal Protective

Bone Metabolism

Thromboxanes (TX)

Platelet Functioning

Vasoconstriction

Leukotrienes (LT)

Mediates inflammation

Immune Regulator

Muscle Contraction

Mucus secretion

Chart 3

The Impact of One Eicosanoid & Enzyme

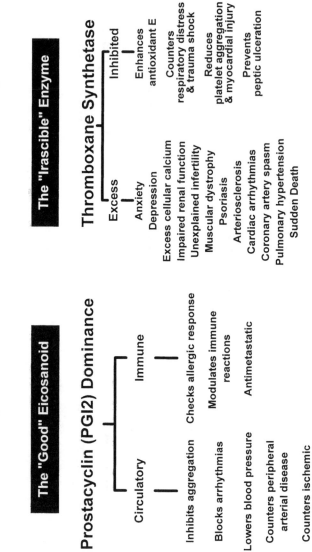

The "Good" Eicosanoid

Prostacyclin (PGI2) Dominance

Circulatory
Inhibits aggregation
Blocks arrhythmias
Lowers blood pressure
Counters peripheral arterial disease
Counters ischemic strokes

Immune
Checks allergic response
Modulates immune reactions
Antimetastatic

The "Irascible" Enzyme

Thromboxane Synthetase

Excess
Anxiety
Depression
Excess cellular calcium
Impaired renal function
Unexplained infertility
Muscular dystrophy
Psoriasis
Arteriosclerosis
Cardiac arrhythmias
Coronary artery spasm
Pulmonary hypertension
Sudden Death

Inhibited
Enhances antioxidant E
Counters respiratory distress & trauma shock
Reduces platelet aggregation & myocardial injury
Prevents peptic ulceration

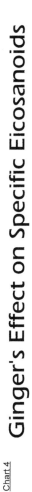

Ginger's Effect on Specific Eicosanoids

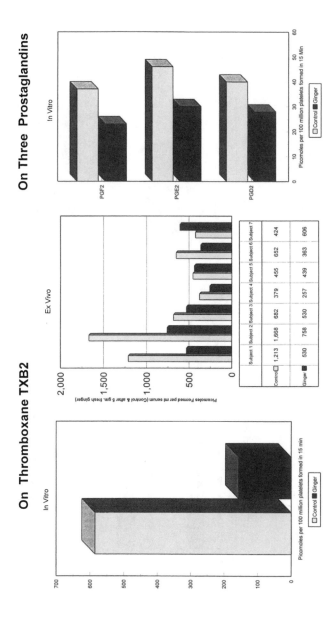

Chart 4

On Three Prostaglandins

In Vitro

PGF2

PGE2

PGD2

0   10   20   30   40   50   60

Picomoles per 100 million platelets formed in 15 Min

☐ Control ■ Ginger

On Thromboxane TXB2

Ex Vivo

2,000

1,500

1,000

500

0

Picomoles Formed per ml serum (Control & after 5 gm. fresh ginger)

	Subject 1	Subject 2	Subject 3	Subject 4	Subject 5	Subject 6	Subject 7
Control ☐	1,213	1,668	682	379	455	652	424
Ginger ■	530	758	530	257	439	363	606

In Vitro

700

600

500

400

300

200

100

0

Picomoles per 100 million platelets formed in 15 min

☐ Control ■ Ginger

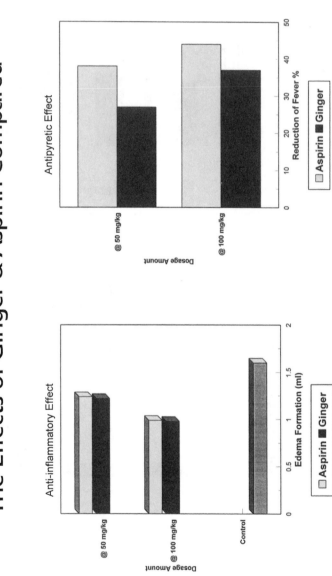

Chart 5

The Effects of Ginger & Aspirin Compared

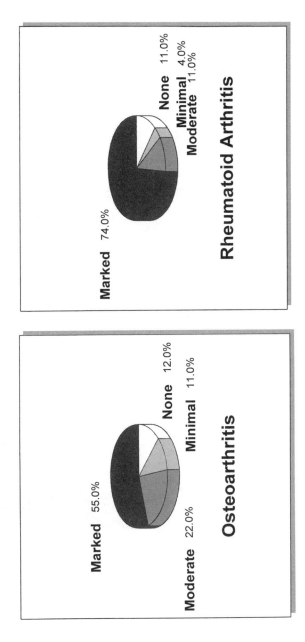

Ginger, Arthritis & Pain Relief

Rheumatoid Arthritis

None 11.0%
Minimal 4.0%
Moderate 11.0%
Marked 74.0%

Osteoarthritis

None 12.0%
Minimal 11.0%
Moderate 22.0%
Marked 55.0%

Chart 6

Chart 7

The Antioxidant Properties of Ginger

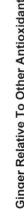

Synergy of Plant Constituents

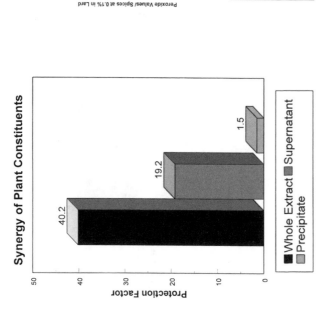

Protection Factor

40.2

19.2

1.5

■ Whole Extract ■ Supernatant
■ Precipitate

Ginger Relative To Other Antioxidants

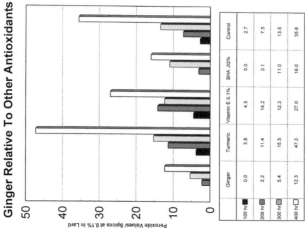

Peroxide Values/ Spices at 0.1% in Lard

	Ginger	Turmeric	Vitamin E 0.1%	BHA .02%	Control
■ 100 hr	0.0	3.8	4.5	0.0	2.7
■ 200 hr	2.2	11.4	14.2	3.1	7.3
■ 300 hr	5.4	16.3	12.3	11.0	13.5
□ 400 hr	12.3	47.3	27.0	16.0	35.6

Ginger's Effects on Digestive Function

Chart 8

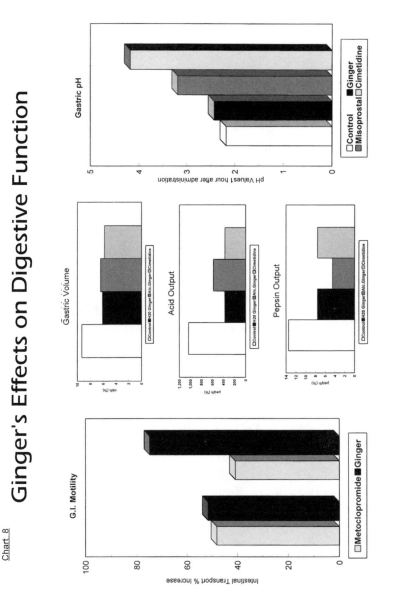

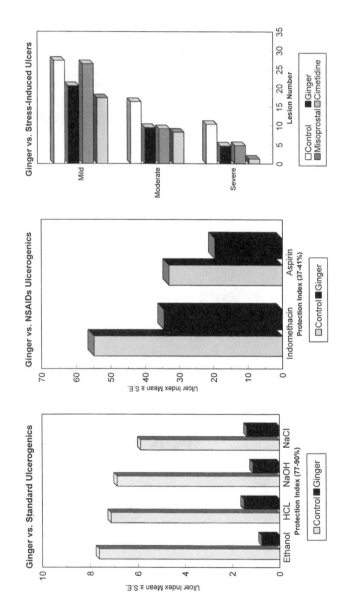

Chart 9

The Ulcer-Protective Spectrum of Ginger

Chart 10

The Twenty Top Selling Drugs for 1992

Rank	Brand Name	Product Type	Marketer	U.S.$ Millions
1	Zantac	Antiulcer agent	Glaxo Inc.	$1,734.60
2	Procardia line	Antihypertensive/anti-anginal	Pfizer Inc.	$1,100.00
3	Mevacor	Cholesterol reducer	Merck & Co., Inc.	$1,040.00
4	Cardizem line	Antihypertensive/antianginal	Marion Merrell Dow Inc.	$ 922.00
5	Vasotec	Antihypertensive	Merck & Co., Inc.	$ 835.00
6	Prozac	Antidepressant	Eli Lilly and Co.	$ 835.00
7	Tagamet	Antiulcer agent	SmithKline Beecham	$ 647.50
8	Ceclor	Anti-infective	Eli Lilly and Co.	$ 640.00
9	Seldane	Antihistamine	Marion Merrell Dow Inc.	$ 614.00
10	Naprosyn	Antiarthritic/analgesic	Syntex Corp.	$ 609.80
11	Cipro	Anti-infective	Miles Inc.	$ 605.00
12	Capoten	Antihypertensive	Bristol-Myers Squibb Co.	$ 598.00
13	Xanax	Antianxiety medicine	The Upjohn Co.	$ 545.00
14	Epogen	Erythropoiesis enhancer	Amgen Inc.	$ 506.30
15	Premarin	Estrogen replacement therapy	Wyeth-Ayerst Labs	$ 505.00
16	Calan line	Antihypertensive/anti-anginal	G.D. Searle & Co.	$ 452.00
17	Pepcid	Antiulcer agent	Merck & Co., Inc.	$ 440.00
18	Lopid	Cholesterol reducer	Warner-Lambert Co.	$ 427.00
19	Proventil	Bronchodilator	Schering-Plough Corp.	$ 426.00
20	Neupogen	Biological response modifier	Amgen Inc.	$ 422.20

Ginger & The Male Reproductive System

Chart 11

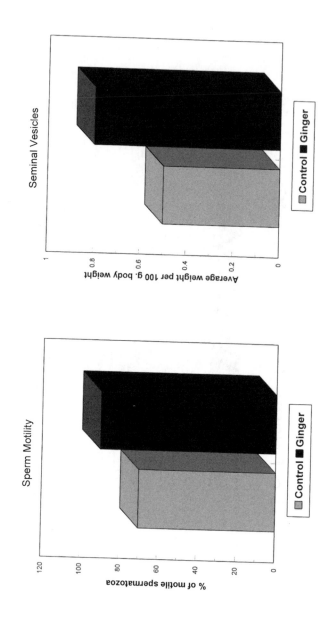

7

GIVE ME MY GINGER

Quality Is Everything

It is quality rather than quantity that matters.
LUCIUS ANNAEUS SENECA, 4 B.C.– A.D. 65

❧NOTE❧
As the well-known adage cited above demonstrates,
quality is an ageless issue. In the case of ginger it
can determine whether one derives benefit or not.

The first concern for those who supplement their diet with
ginger should be the quality of the original rhizome. Ginger
can be valuable in many forms; however, if the original
starting material is old, shriveled, moldy or chemically
treated, it will obviously not yield the same values as a
product created from a fresh, organically grown rhizome.

To insure an international supply of top-quality ginger
products, an extensive grading system has been developed: for example, governments like the United Kingdom
and Canada have set exacting standards for fresh and
dried ginger, essential oils and oleoresin. Unfortunately,
one of the issues which needs greater attention is that of

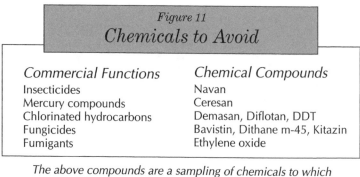

Figure 11
Chemicals to Avoid

Commercial Functions	Chemical Compounds
Insecticides	Navan
Mercury compounds	Ceresan
Chlorinated hydrocarbons	Demasan, Diflotan, DDT
Fungicides	Bavistin, Dithane m-45, Kitazin
Fumigants	Ethylene oxide

The above compounds are a sampling of chemicals to which commercial ginger can be exposed. To avoid these potentially toxic chemicals, it is highly recommended that one request, before purchasing a ginger supplement, a company's allowable chemical limits or organic certification. This standard should also apply to the naturally occuring aflatoxin mold.

chemical exposure. During cultivation, storage and processing, ginger can be barraged with chemicals, including mercury compounds, chlorinated hydrocarbons, fungicides and fumigants[1]♦ *(see figure 11).*

Ultimately, the opportunity to examine the fresh ginger rhizome and review it for chemical exposure before processing it into powder or finished products would be ideal. Considering that in most cases this would be a very difficult or impossible process, one's first choice should be to seek out an organic product that has been certified through any number of state and international organizations like OVONA and OCIA. This is especially important for people who are interested in taking larger amounts of ginger for therapeutic reasons.

♦ Natural fungal toxins like aflatoxins have also been reported to contaminate ginger.

Snap or Extract

✦NOTE✧

Things would be much easier if there were only one
type of ginger product to recommend. Fortunately
for the consumer, it can be argued that benefit can
be gained from them all. One cannot go wrong with
the following recommendation: Consume ginger in
both the fresh and dry forms, if possible.

Starting with fresh or dry rhizome, ginger is processed into
a myriad of finished forms including syrups, candies, jams,
capsules, extracts, liqueurs, pickles, cookies and beer, to
name a few. If Cornell researchers noticed that a ginger
marmalade could have had such a dramatic impact on
platelet aggregation, then the therapeutic principles are
obviously quite stable or resistant to processing. Therefore,
it is fair to say that each finished form has its own distinct
advantages. Candied forms, for example, might be objected
to because of the presence of sucrose but if a choice is to be
made between an artificially flavored and colored confec-
tion and a candy with an actual health potential, the choice
is clear. Besides, the candied form actually gives ginger a
wider, more mainstream audience to offer benefit, including
people who might never have considered taking ginger as a
health supplement. This same principle obviously holds true
for beers, cookies and other popular foods.

To receive two of the best-researched therapeutic constituent groups of ginger, the gingerols (fresh) and
shogaols (dry), it is reasonable to assert that a combination of ginger products is best. Depending upon the processing methods, different products will have varying
levels of these two critical groups.✦ As detailed in *figure
12*, gingerols and shogaols each have their own health

✦ Roasted ginger may have pronounced advantages over dried ginger in preventing ulcers.

Figure 12
Gingerols and Shogaols: Confirmed Actions & Effects

	Gingerols	Shogaols
Principal Action[□]		
Anti-5HT3	*[2] □	
Lipoxygenase inhibition	*[3]	
Prostaglandin inhibition	*[4]	
Observed Effect		
Analgesic	*[5]	*<
Anthelmintic	*>[6]	*
Anticathartic	*[7]	*<
Antiemetic	*[8]	*<[9]
Antifungal	*[10]	
Antihepatotoxic	*[11]	*
Antipyretic	*[5]	*<
Antitussive	*[13]	*[12]
Antiulcer	*[15]	*[14]
Cardiotonic	*[16]	
G.I. Motility	*[16]	
Hypotensive	*[5]	*<
Thermoregulatory	*>[17]	*

* The absence of a star does not mean that the group is necessarily without that action or effect. It could mean that it is not yet confirmed.

□ [8]-Gingerol more potent than [6] or [10]

> and < indicate which of the two constituents was found to be stronger.

The approximately twelve-member team of gingerols and shogaols is widely recognized as the generals leading the army of ginger's therapeutic principles. Whereas the gingerols have been credited with virtually all of ginger's properties, the above figure clearly demonstrates that the shogaols (abundant in dried ginger) are an equally important and potent force.

advantages. For example, the gingerols are more potent as antihepatotoxics[18] and anthelmintics,[19] while the shogaols appear to be more effective as anti-inflammatory agents, antipyretics and analgesics.[20]

The individual value of each ginger product is confirmed in traditional Oriental medicine where four different forms of ginger–fresh, dried, steamed and roasted– are actually considered separate drugs, each prescribed for a specific group of applications.[20]♦ To alleviate the concern that one needs to consume every conceivable ginger product to gain benefit, one Chinese study suggests that all the forms have more in common than one would suspect. Of twenty-five studied elements, there was only a maximum variation of three novel or missing constituents.[21]

Four Basics

❧NOTE❧

The enormous variety of finished ginger products can be fitted into four major categories. They are fresh, dried, syruped-candied and extracted. The following offers an overview of each form's applications and advantages. The section "For Health and Against Disease" deals with dosages.

Get Fresh

Whatever the final form, it is easy to argue that there is an intangible advantage to the fresh rhizome. The flavor of fresh ginger is itself a study in culinary art *(see figure 13)*. This is underlined by a recent fragrance test which noted that fresh ginger can be recognized for its scent at a dilution as low as 1 part in 35,000, while powdered ginger is only 1 part in 1,500-2,000.[22] The fresh form can be used in many different applications from hot compresses and culinary spice to medicinal tea.

♦ To those who use or prescribe herbs, one has to wonder to what degree other plants undergo significant transformations during processing. In promotional literature one might hear that one form of an herb is better than another. However, the story of ginger reveals that each could possess its own range of distinct positive effects.

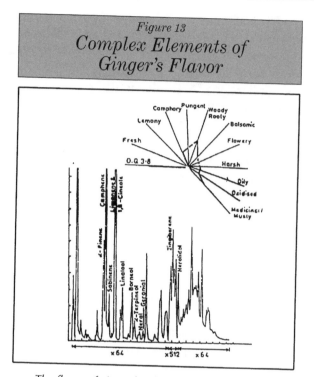

Figure 13
Complex Elements of Ginger's Flavor

The flavor of ginger has been extensively studied throughout the world. The two images above, presented in CRC Critical Reviews, each outline particular aspects of what gives ginger its distinctive flavor. The top image is a subjective taste rating score associated with the lower gas chromatogram. When the two are combined, a signature profile can be given to a ginger sample.[23]

It is understandable why anyone who has ever used a ginger compress names it as one of their most precious health routines. Among myriad applications, a ginger compress is remarkably effective for virtually all external signs of inflammatory processes including muscular stiffness and headaches. It is also a most valuable healing remedy for swollen glands, chest and head colds and stomach cramps. To use as a compress, follow the instructions detailed in *figure 14*.

Ginger tea is the perfect after-dinner drink, fasting staple, weight-loss aid and pain or cold remedy *(see figure*

Figure 14
Yamoda Ginger Compress

While bringing a gallon of distilled or spring water to boil in a large, lidded enamel pot, wash 1½ fresh, unpeeled ginger rhizomes and grate by hand using a rotating, clockwise motion. This keeps tough fibers from building up on the grater.

Place the grated ginger in a clean muslin cloth, slightly moistened, and tie at top to form a bag, leaving room inside for air and water to circulate.

Before dropping this bag into the pot, gently squeeze the juice from the bag into the water, which should no longer be boiling.

Cover pot and simmer for 7 minutes.

The resulting liquid should have a golden hue and a distinctive ginger aroma.

When ready, remove pot from stove and set aside.

When the liquid is still hot but not scalding, dip a terry cloth hand towel into it and apply directly to site of pain.

The compress should be kept fairly warm for 15 to 20 minutes. Repeat again 4 to 6 hours later.

This remedy of Dr. Koji Yamoda is said to relieve a wide variety of external and internal pains including neuralgia, stiffness, swollen glands and toothache. A ginger compress is reported to be effective for patients suffering from asthma and bronchitis. Consult with your holistic physician when treating serious disorders.[24]

15). To make a tea, place approximately ½ teaspoon of freshly grated rhizome into 8 ounces of boiling water, cover pot and steep for 10 to 15 minutes, allowing full extraction of the fresh rhizome. Strain and add honey to taste. ginger also makes an excellent tonifying iced tea.

Adding fresh ginger to the diet can be done in a wonderful variety of ways. One of my favorites is to simply add it as part of a daily juicing routine including carrot and apple. Be careful to gradually add the fresh ginger juice to your routine gradually as it is quite potent.♦ To

---

♦ An interesting side note: it is a traditional practice in the Middle East and particularly Saudi Arabia to add ginger to coffee. I have heard from coffee drinkers here in the U.S. that by doing this they require less coffee to deliver its stimulating properties. Considering ginger's principal stimulant and bioavailability actions, these observed effects are not surprising. To mix ginger with coffee, one can simply add powdered or fresh grated ginger into the preperked coffee grounds. An alternative would be to add the alcohol extract described above to the already brewed coffee. I offer this simply as a point of information and not as an endorsement of coffee drinking.

discover some of the best ginger recipes, an excellent resource is Bruce Cost's book *Ginger East to West*.

Certainly the Sweetest

Candied ginger ranks as one of the world's most popular confections. Processed with fresh ginger and sucrose, it can be a convenient form for taking ginger while traveling or as a delightful and effective after-dinner digestive aid. *Ginger East to West* contains an easy recipe for making candied or crystallized ginger.

A honey-based syrup offers an even more desirable means to deliver the health benefits of ginger. Honey has a long history of being used to deliver the therapeutic values of herbs, and ginger is no exception. Dating back to the sixth-century A.D., a recipe is described for a ginger-honey syrup. The recipe appears in a manual with a telling title: *Essential Arts for the Equalization of the People.*[25]

Honey offers its own range of excellent synergistic values to ginger, especially if the ginger can be low-heat-infused into the honey.♦ Besides enhancing the flavor, preservation, and variety of applications for a ginger product, honey possesses its own range of antibacterial,[27] anticancer,[28] antifungal,[29] wound-healing,[30] and antiulcer[31] properties. A book similar to this one could easily be written on honey itself, but a few points deserve mention here related to ginger.

While honey broadens ginger's antibacterial and antifungal benefits, combined with ginger it also enhances its antiulcer properties. Honey is protective to the gastric mucosa[32] and shows significant activity against Helicobacter pylori,[33] the species associated with peptic ulcers. For those people concerned about a potential conflict between honey and blood sugar or candida albicans treatment programs, evidence suggests that honey is significantly better tolerated than commonly used simple sugars like sucrose.[34] A factor in honey is also found active against candida albicans.[35]

♦ Unfortunately, the boiling of both the ginger and the honey in the traditional Chinese recipe presents some issues in the final product. Above 160° Fahrenheit, one of the key enzymes in ginger, zingibain, is inactivated as well as some of the enzymes in honey. Traditional Ayurvedic medicine also advises against cooking honey.

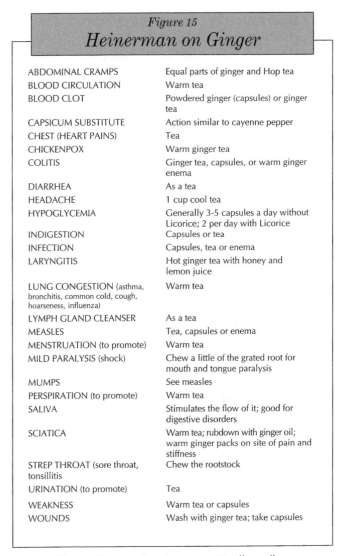

Figure 15

Heinerman on Ginger

ABDOMINAL CRAMPS	Equal parts of ginger and Hop tea
BLOOD CIRCULATION	Warm tea
BLOOD CLOT	Powdered ginger (capsules) or ginger tea
CAPSICUM SUBSTITUTE	Action similar to cayenne pepper
CHEST (HEART PAINS)	Tea
CHICKENPOX	Warm ginger tea
COLITIS	Ginger tea, capsules, or warm ginger enema
DIARRHEA	As a tea
HEADACHE	1 cup cool tea
HYPOGLYCEMIA	Generally 3-5 capsules a day without Licorice; 2 per day with Licorice
INDIGESTION	Capsules or tea
INFECTION	Capsules, tea or enema
LARYNGITIS	Hot ginger tea with honey and lemon juice
LUNG CONGESTION (asthma, bronchitis, common cold, cough, hoarseness, influenza)	Warm tea
LYMPH GLAND CLEANSER	As a tea
MEASLES	Tea, capsules or enema
MENSTRUATION (to promote)	Warm tea
MILD PARALYSIS (shock)	Chew a little of the grated root for mouth and tongue paralysis
MUMPS	See measles
PERSPIRATION (to promote)	Warm tea
SALIVA	Stimulates the flow of it; good for digestive disorders
SCIATICA	Warm tea; rubdown with ginger oil; warm ginger packs on site of pain and stiffness
STREP THROAT (sore throat, tonsillitis	Chew the rootstock
URINATION (to promote)	Tea
WEAKNESS	Warm tea or capsules
WOUNDS	Wash with ginger tea; take capsules

*The applications for ginger are virtually endless.
John Heinerman is a medical anthropologist and author of
numerous articles and texts on herbs. Heinerman's suggested
uses for ginger are included here to exemplify a few of these
applications and forms.*[36]

*(Reprinted with permission from **The Complete Book of Spices,**
by John Heinerman, published by Keats Publishing, Inc.,
New Canaan, Conn.)*

In addition to the ginger-and-honey combination, a health tonic or cough/cold syrup,♦ ginger-and-honey can be used as a hot beverage or tea sweetener, cooking seasoning or table sauce, dessert topping or mixed with carbonated water to create a delicious homemade ginger ale.

To produce your own ginger syrup, add one part of fresh ginger, grated or juiced, to three parts of honey and refrigerate (be sure to peel the ginger rhizome to extend its values and prevent fermentation.) Generally one to two teaspoons will be appropriate per 8 ounces of carbonated or hot water.

Sweet Route to Heading Off Colon Cancer

In recent years, a host of studies have identified a broad spectrum of medical attributes in honey–including antifungal, antibacterial, anti-inflammatory, antiproliferative, and cancer-drug-potentiating properties. Now, researchers at the American Health Foundation in Valhalla, N.Y., have uncovered another. In the September 15 issue of *Cancer Research*, Bandaru S. Reddy and his co-workers describe the ability of honey-derived caffeic esters to inhibit the development of precancerous changes in the colon of rats given a known carcinogen. These esters come from the propolis—the brown, resinous, tree-derived material that honeybees use to cement together their hives. Reddy's group considers three derivatives of the caffeic esters promising enough to use in the longer-term animal studies of colon cancer.

SCIENCE NEWS 1993 [37]

From Tablespoon to Tub

One of the most versatile and powerful ways to experience the benefits of ginger is as a dehydrated powder. In this form one can obtain two principal values: 1) up to ten times the concentration of certain fresh ginger elements; and 2) novel therapeutic compounds. Powdered ginger

---

♦ To maximize the syrup's antitussive properties, powdered ginger should be included in the formulation.

will have more nutrients because of the removal of moisture, but more importantly it will possess high levels of shogaols, which, as stated earlier, are reported to possess more of ginger's significant aspirin-like qualities.

After a high-quality source has been verified, powdered ginger can be effectively used both internally and externally. Powdered ginger can be used in many of the same applications as the fresh form including compresses, as a tea and in cooking. Taken in capsules, or by the teaspoon in food or in liquid, this form provides the anti-inflammatory benefits and an excellent spectrum of digestive, cardiovascular tonic-protectant properties. Used externally in compresses or in baths, ginger powder provides powerful, stimulating, transdermal and aromatherapeutic effects. Ginger powder is excellent as a moistened chest compress or added by the tablespoon to a hot bath for relief of muscle strains and cold symptoms. To make a chest compress with powdered ginger simply moisten 2-3 teaspoons with hot water and spread over a hot, wet cotton towel. If skin is sensitive, use less and build up slowly. Ginger capsules and bulk powder are readily available nationwide in natural-food stores.

Alcohol's Bright Side

Alcohol is recognized traditionally and in modern research as an excellent extraction agent for the properties of herbs. A double-macerated or highly potent alcohol extract of dried ginger can deliver all the benefits of this form including significant levels of beneficial shogaols. To maximize or balance the benefits of this alcohol extract, fresh ginger juice can be added. This addition serves a dual purpose; while it complements the dried with its unique fresh elements like gingerols, it lowers the final alcohol concentration to a level that most people should well tolerate.

The principal benefits of the extracted form are convenience and concentration. Within seconds a dropper of the

extract, taken straight◆ or in a glass of water, will deliver
the full range of ginger's dried and fresh benefits.
Although it is not as practical to use the extract in cooking or compresses, as a therapeutic form it offers the
most immediate and powerful therapeutic response for
the treatment of digestive disorders or cold symptoms.⌐

> Alcohol and acetone have been generally used for extrac-
> tion of the [ginger] oleoresin. Both solvents give satisfac-
> tory oleoresins although the yield with alcohol is reported
> to be higher, in some cases as much as three times.
> V.S. GOVINDARAJAN[38]

◆ Those who are unfamiliar with the pungency of ginger should always begin taking the
extract diluted in water.

⌐ A 1-ounce bottle of equal parts fresh juice and 1:1 extract of dried rhizome represents
approximately 1 ounce of fresh rhizome and ½ ounce dried rhizome. The ½ ounce of extract
from dried ginger is actually equivalent to approximately 5 ounces of fresh rhizome. This cal-
culation is based upon a ratio of 10 pounds of fresh being necessary to produce 1 pound of
dried and 2 pounds of fresh rhizome to make 16 fluid ounces of fresh juice. Assuming this 1-
ounce bottle contains a total of 480 drops and that a 2-milliliter dropper is 32 drops. Keep in
mind that different droppers have different openings and therefore will yield different drop
sizes. For example, a small dropper might yield as many as 1,100 drops per 1 ounce bottle
thereby requiring more than double the drops. The reason the extract form is the most potent
is that the fiber has been removed allowing immediate benefit.

For Health and against Disease

❧NOTE❧

And now the most frequently asked question: How much ginger should I take? Taking into consideration an almost infinite variety of circumstances, recommendations for using ginger are made. With the exception of serious health problems, in which case a holistic health practitioner's advice is suggested, there is ample room for experimentation.

Upon reaching this point one is naturally inclined to ask the most obvious and ultimately challenging question: How much ginger should I take? One can extend the process of answering this question to amazing detail considering literally dozens of variables like intended use, one's age, medical history and genetic makeup and the quality and nature of the product. Fortunately, unlike virtually every modern drug, one will have difficulty erring on the high, or overdose, side. One of ginger's most convincing testimonials is its multi-millennia safety record. The historical literature contains virtually no mention of adverse effects and the body of modern scientific literature supports this with a unanimous verdict of: *no side effects (see the section "Safety First" on page 87)*. With this consideration in mind, one is therefore most likely to err by taking too little or by selecting an improper or low-quality form.

Taking into account the above qualifiers and the body of historical and modern research, an attempt is made here to offer broad guidelines to the reader. The four basic forms are therefore broken down into two major categories: how to use ginger for health and against disease. Needless to say, for both categories, it is recommended that one always consider the synergistic value of other herbs and healing modalities.

Figure 16
Ginger for Health

Form of Ginger	Minimum Daily Suggested Intake
Dried rhizome ^	1,000 milligrams
Fresh rhizome *	1 teaspoon grated
Liquid extract o	2 droppers (2 milliliters)
Syrup	2 teaspoons (10 milliliters)

^This number represents the approximate dosage suggested by Israeli researcher Backon and that defined by Danish researcher Srivastava and one-fifth of the intake described by Indian researcher Verma. Professor Srivastava recommends after observation of benefits reducing the daily dosage to 500 milligrams.

*One teaspoon of fresh grated ginger rhizome weighs approximately 7 grams.

°Each dropper represents approximately 1,865 milligrams of fresh and 931 milligrams of dried rhizome. If one adds one part of juice to three parts of honey, two teaspoons of syrup represent approximately 2.5 milliliters of fresh juice. Approximately 125 milligrams of dried rhizome can easily be added to a teaspoon of the syrup, increasing its pungency and efficacy.

These quantities offer minimum intake guidelines for the general public in order to obtain benefit from ginger.

For Health

Figure 16 suggests very broad dosage guidelines for the general population to gain the tonic and preventive benefits of ginger. To some extent, what one expects to gain from ginger will determine how much and when it is taken. For example, to enhance digestion of a meal or the effects of dietary supplements, simply take ginger at mealtime or ten to fifteen minutes before and after eating. For the beneficial effects on the circulatory system, specifically the antiplatelet aggregation effect, the research suggests that it might take up to seven days and/or dosages in excess of 2 grams powdered rhizome for maximum result.♦ For prevention of nausea or vomiting,

♦ Recently published research in England (Lumb 1994),[39] suggests that a dosage of under 2 grams and less than 24 hours will either be an inadequate dosage or time duration to notice an antiplatelet aggregation effect. Research in India (Verma 1993) demonstrated that 5 grams, taken for seven days, show a significant effect. Interestingly, Lumb conducted the study to affirm that ginger, used successfully as an antiemetic before surgery, would not interfere with normal platelet function.

as mentioned earlier, one would want to start dosing with a minimum of 1,000 milligrams at least three hours prior to a challenging event. For general tonic benefits, one of the best ways to begin a day is with a glass of ginger tea or homemade ginger ale.

One might want to take increased amounts or a variety of the different forms to enhance one's range of benefits. Still, as a commonsense precaution, it is important that the intake be gradual and that there be no observations of ill effects. There is not necessarily a best time to take ginger. Some people like the warming sensation of ginger on an empty stomach, while others find this experience uncomfortable. If one should experience discomfort, then simply decrease the dosage, take with other foods and, particularly at the beginning, drink plenty of juice or water with the ginger.♦

Against Disease

Using ginger as part of a disease treatment program is an obviously more involved process and requires greater explanation. In an attempt to simplify this, health conditions are broken down into two categories: self-limiting and potentially life-threatening.

The self-limiting category includes conditions like minor infections and localized inflammatory processes. In this class are those ailments for which most over-the-counter drugs are prescribed. As a broad guideline for this grouping, ginger should be able to be used liberally and obviously with far less concern for side effects than commercial compounds. Just as one would take two tablets of aspirin every two to three hours for a headache, a minimum of 1,000 milligrams of dried ginger could be substituted. As with the guidelines previously mentioned in the section "*For Health*," fresh, powder, extract or syrup can be used

---

♦ Although I have never read it in the literature, it is possible that some people might experience an allergic reaction to some of the commercial processing agents used to create many of the popular ginger products. If you are using a noncertified organic product, be aware of additives like sulfur dioxide or possible pesticide residues.

interchangeably as long as fresh and dry equivalents are given. It is comforting to know that ginger has a decided advantage over modern pharmaceuticals in that there is a substantial opportunity for experimentation.

In the case of serious or life-threatening health conditions, it is advised that the treatment protocol be guided by the patient's holistic health practitioner. This advice is noted for three principal reasons: 1) there needs to be more human research with clear dosage guidelines; 2) there are so many different medical conditions, some with an obviously great need for monitoring; and 3) ginger, especially in large doses, might affect the bioavailability of other therapeutic aids and either intensify or negate aspects of their effectiveness.

When working in this class with your practitioner, request that your doctor review this book. For example, in the case of rheumatoid arthritis, you and your physician could consider the daily dosage and observation of benefits mentioned in the Srivastava studies. Although the suggested dosage by the authors was 500–1,000 milligrams, subjects who consumed three or more times this suggested dose (approximately 3 to 7 grams of powdered rhizome) reported better and quicker relief of symptoms. Some of the most dramatic results were noted when patients consumed as much as 50 grams of fresh rhizome. Keep in mind that ginger is not a cure for arthritis. Srivastava noted in his studies that when subjects discontinued their ginger supplementation, symptoms returned. This highlights the need to include other holistic protocols such as dietary modification and stress reduction in the treatment of arthritis.

For some of the other principal conditions described in this book, such as ulcers or cardiovascular disease, animal studies suggest a similarly wide range. Keep in mind that there are no human studies delineating how to use ginger to treat ulcers or specific heart conditions, so treatment should definitely be undertaken only under the guidance of a holistic physician. Regarding ulcers, keep in mind that although there might be an experience of initial gastric irritation, research and testimonials on other pungent botanicals like cayenne pepper and the antiulcer research on ginger suggest that the initial discomfort may be both acceptable and necessary. Experiment to determine your own best routine, exploring with your physician the potential of other synergistic botanicals like licorice root and hawthorn berry and leaf.

As to when one might observe benefits, the range might be from immediate (as in treating intestinal gas or headache) to as long as one to three months for more chronic conditions. If apparent benefits are slow in coming, it is reassuring to remember that while one system is being healed, others are likewise being balanced or protected. Again, no modern drug can make this claim so confidently or safely.

It must be restated that when ginger is used in a disease treatment program or in larger doses, it is advised that the fresh-dry equivalents be defined and that the product have some type of quality assurance as to levels of foreign chemicals.

Safety First

During the 2.5-year period of ginger consumption, no side effects were reported.
K. C. SRIVASTAVA[40]

As tempting as it might be to say that there is no limit to daily ginger dosage–especially in light of the 50-gram quantities consumed in some studies with no side effects and its historically liberal consumption even as a vegetable–common sense dictates that upper limits must exist.

In attempting to define an upper or safety limit for ginger, there are three areas that justify mention and prudence. Keep in mind that the following information is theoretical and there are no specific studies to support these concerns.

First, since ginger is a modulator of eicosanoids and can inhibit thromboxanes, Joshua Backon alerts regular consumers that blood-clotting times after surgery might be affected. Backon specifically raises this concern before wholeheartedly endorsing ginger supplementation for nausea after gynecological surgery. The work of the English researcher Lumb suggests that as long as two grams of powdered rhizome in a twenty-four-hour period are not exceeded, there should be no reason for concern.

The second related reservation regarding ginger is consumption during pregnancy, specifically in the first trimester.♦ Ginger has historically been used as an emmenagogue and in large doses as an abortifacient, although in the latter case, the dosage is not clearly defined. If one weighs this historical application with research findings stating that ginger is statistically effective and safe for the nausea of pregnancy,[41] my conclusion is simply that moderation or prudence should be exercised. As a conservative safety guideline, during the first trimester and before parturition, it is advised that dosages used in the Fischer-Rasmussen study (1,000 milligrams dried rhizome) should either not be exceeded or be increased very gradually under a physician's guidance. Although exact equivalents to the dry are difficult or impossible to determine because of the different constituents in fresh and dry rhizome and the varying quality of commercial preparations, it is advised that the minimum daily suggested intakes in *figure 16* be used as the maximum guideline for all finished forms.

Last, as mentioned previously, if you are taking prescription drugs, consult with your physician before beginning the consumption of more than the conservative guidelines described above. It is quite possible that ginger might mediate or negate the activity of certain prescriptions.

> Some of the patients with arthritic disorders who
> mistakenly took 3-4 times, or even more, the
> dose (0.5-1.0 gram powdered ginger/day) suggested by us,
> reported quicker and better [arthritis] relief than those
> on the recommended dose.
> K. C. SRIVASTAVA[42]

♦ Regarding lactation, one source reports that it is well known in Jamaica that ginger can reduce a lactating mother's milk flow. [43] This can be either a benefit or a detriment, depending on the desire of the mother.

8

FREEDOM AND HEALTH AT THE CROSSROADS

❦❦❦❦

The Real Crises

If you're feeling well, just stay away from the doctor.
EUGENE ROBBINS, M.D., PROFESSOR EMERITUS,
STANFORD UNIVERSITY[1]

___❦NOTE❦___

There is probably only one consensus regarding modern health care: The system is in crisis. Before we can see how ginger might fit into this mind-boggling puzzle, the true problem needs to be clearly identified. The crisis lies not in the need for more or cheaper doctors and drugs, but in the flawed precepts of modern medicine. It is this deep conceptual fault that is challenging both our financial and physical well-being.

Death by Prescription

More than 50 percent of the average American diet consists of processed foods that contain some 3,000 different food additives. The typical American ingests fifteen pounds of these food additives each year.[2] Every hour 660,000 animals are killed for meat in the United States,[3] and every three days the average American consumes a pound of white sugar. In 1982, the National Research Council determined that diet was "probably the greatest single factor in the epidemic of cancer, particularly for cancers of the breast, colon and prostate."[4]

> Despite an all-out war on cancer over the past
> 20 years, people are developing malignancies at a
> higher rate than ever before.
> *SCIENCE NEWS 1994*[5]

    The currently prevailing health-care system is unfortunately incapable of changing this direction. Instead of remedying the underlying reasons why so many of us are sick, the system is structured simply to bandage the problem or manage disease.

    Studies show that more doctors or more physicals are hardly the answers. The Kaiser Permanente Health Group in California reported no significant difference in death rates for people who did or did not receive physicals.[6]

    We certainly don't need more surgery. More harm than good has been demonstrated by many commonly performed procedures. For example, men who receive radical prostate surgery experience incontinence and impotence rates from the surgery itself of 30 and 90 percent respectively. Men who avoid this surgical procedure are found to benefit more from "watchful waiting." The researcher, Dr. John Wasson, concluded in a study published in the *Journal of the American Medical Association* (*JAMA*) that "we have, in essence, an epidemic of treatment and no scientific proof that it's valid. The take-home message is that we don't know what we're doing, but we're doing a lot of it."[7]

    Last, no one really believes we need more prescription drugs. By the time we Americans are age fifty, almost one out of three of us will be on eight or more prescription drugs[8] and, according to recent figures cited in *JAMA*, between 60,000 to 140,000 of us will die each year from adverse reactions to these drugs.[9]

51.5 percent of drugs approved by the FDA have serious
post-approval risks including heart failure, birth defects,
kidney failure, blindness and convulsions.

1990 GAO REPORT [10]

The Money Pit

To add irony to agony, our current disease-care system is
killing us financially. Our total health-care bill is a staggering $3 billion daily, the highest of all industrialized nations.
Included in this bill is an excessive 800 percent markup for
the pharmaceutical industry's adverse-effect-riddled drugs.

The consequences of maintaining this faltering system
are already devastating to business and middle-class
America. Health-care costs are the leading reason for
bankruptcy, and one million Americans earning $25,000 to
50,000 annually lost their health insurance last year alone
due to inflated premium costs.[11] Recognizing the peril of
this crisis at a recent conference on health care, President
Clinton banged a table with his fist and told the 300 par-
ticipants that "the cost of health care is a joke. It is going
to bankrupt this country." [12] Considering the tragic fact
that among industrialized nations, we place close to the
lowest in life expectancy (fifteenth) and highest in all cancer and heart disease rates, it is painfully obvious that
our national health system is chronically ill — not to mention a very bad investment.

We don't know what we're doing in medicine. Perhaps
one-quarter to one-third of medical services may be of little or no benefit to patients.

DR. DAVID EDDY, DIRECTOR, DUKE UNIVERSITY
HEALTH POLICY RESEARCH [13]

The scientific basis of medicine is much weaker than most
patients or even physicians realize; this leads to treatment
based on uncertainty.

C. EVERETT KOOP, M.D.,
FORMER U.S. SURGEON GENERAL [14]

Milligrams of Hope

The evidence is accumulating that people who are taking
an antioxidant of some sort seem to have a high degree of
protection from coronary heart disease.

Dr. Claude Lenfant, Director of the
National Heart, Lung and Blood Institute [15]

*NOTE*

When considering this nation's and more broadly the
world's health-care crisis, our story on ginger is
seemingly insignificant. But, when appreciated for
its far-reaching healing and political potential, this
report takes on fantastic proportions. Ginger, at
once common and superlative, can trigger a dramatic
change in the way the industrialized world views
medicine. This change would take the form of a
renewed look at the thousands of years of medical
tradition and, specifically, the enormous potential
that less invasive natural healing modalities offer.
Clearly, there are signs that this transformation is
beginning to happen, and the time and conditions
could not be more ripe.

While we are getting poorer and probably sicker as a
nation, there are flickers of hope. New doors are beginning
to open in the renowned edifices of the U.S. health-care
establishment. The most respected medical journals are
now acknowledging that simple changes in diet and the
mere addition of milligrams of dietary supplements hold
the potential for drastically improving the nation's health.

Recently published studies proclaim that we can con-
ceivably disarm two of our greatest killers, heart disease
and cancer, by simply adding to the diet food constituents
like antioxidants beta carotene and vitamin E. Researchers
are going so far as to suggest that dietary supplements like
vitamin E could lower the risk of heart disease, indepen-
dent of other risk factors by as much as 40 to 50 percent.[16]

Noting that heart attacks alone kill 600,000 Americans annually, this safe and easy prescription could potentially save hundreds of thousands of lives and billions of dollars each year. Considering that more powerful antioxidants than vitamin E naturally occur in herbs like ginger,[17] and that many of these herbs are proving therapeutic potentials transcending those of our most powerful drugs,[18] a profound possibility is waiting to be tapped.

Last, rating perhaps as the most positive development, is the recent opening of the Office of Alternative Medicine (OAM) at the National Institutes of Health (NIH). It is hard to believe that the NIH, a bastion of conservative allopathic medicine, has actually opened an office to examine the efficacy of alternative forms of health care like herbal medicine and acupuncture. Although the budget for this office is only one-five-thousandth of that of NIH as a whole, it is a promising sign of events to come.

The Roadblocks

❧NOTE❧

The FDA and the pharmaceutical, food, medical and insurance industries all have deep-rooted investments in the current health-care system. Unfortunately, these investments have collectively manifested to become a veritable Berlin Wall of health, preventing both innovative thought and personal freedoms. This section identifies some of these critical problems and proposes brief solutions.

Herbs like ginger and the traditions of thousands of years of natural healing modalities will never be fully understood, appreciated or allowed to fulfill their mission unless major problems are identified and eliminated in our current health-care system. Needless to say, whole books are written trying to diagnose and answer these problems. Since the focus of this book is on ginger and not the intricacies of our current health-care establishment, this discussion will be brief.

I would not be so foolish or unrealistic as to suggest eliminating the doctors or the drugs or the governmental establishment that has evolved to support them. Rather, I would like to expose a few problems with these modern icons which I label as the roadblocks and propose the most basic and simplest of solutions. Acknowledging the considerable risk of being labeled oversimplistic, I hope there will be some value in this exercise.

The FDA

The American public does not have the knowledge to make wise health-care decisions. . . . Trust us. We will tell you what's good for you.

DAVID KESSLER, FDA COMMISSIONER ON
LARRY KING LIVE, 1992 [19]

THE PROBLEM:

Unfortunately, the agency given the authority to dictate what information is disseminated to the public on foods, drugs and general health claims–the U.S. Food and Drug Administration (FDA)–has held a long bias against preventive health and the natural-foods and dietary-supplement industry.

What is the physiological effect of prunes? How about coffee? Is ginger good for digestion? When I ask these questions of an audience, without exception everyone knows the answers. Strangely and disturbingly, as of this writing, if this truthful information is placed on a product label or even in a brochure, the FDA has determined it to be a violation of the law.

The government agency brings its bias a step further by promoting the notion that herbs and other dietary supplements are inherently dangerous. The FDA refers to safe and soothing teas made with herbs like chamomile as "unknown brews" implying that there are perils lurking within them. *The FDA Consumer*, the agency journal, absurdly depicts herbal teas with a skull and crossbones.[20] Considering that three of the top four causes of lethal poisonings in the U.S. are FDA-approved drugs[21] and that a toxicity category is virtually nonexistent for herbal dietary supplements, the skull-and-cross-bones symbol is clearly misplaced.

To make matters worse, the agency has for the past twenty years continuously attempted through wily, circuitous and one-dimensional arguments to regulate virtually all traditional medicinal or tonic herbs out of the U.S. marketplace, thus threatening both national health and medical freedom of choice.

> FDA's definition is so broad, it would classify every component of food — even single ingredients — as food additives. The only justification for the FDA Alice-in-Wonderland approach is to allow the FDA to make an end run around a statutory scheme.
>
> *JUDGE CUDAHY, U.S. COURT OF APPEALS*
> *7TH CIRCUIT*[22]

THE SOLUTION:

The FDA should appoint a panel of experts who are open-minded and aware of alternative health-care modalities. Fair and clear guidelines should be given, actually encouraging the use and development of safe and inexpensive dietary supplements and traditional medicines. This age-old therapeutic class truly deserves its own regulatory category free of the draconian impediments of modern drug classifications. Also, the structure of the process that results in drug companies spending up to $359 million for drug approval and marketing should be reevaluated. It is hard to imagine how traditional health remedies will be integrated as long as drug companies are spending these huge sums of money.

The Pharmaceutical Industry

> In 1990, the top ten pharmaceutical houses had profit margins three times that of the average Fortune 500 company.... Over the past decade drug prices have risen at almost triple the rate of inflation.
>
> *1990 GAO (GENERAL ACCOUNTING OFFICE) REPORT*[23]

THE PROBLEM:

The pharmaceutical industry is arguably the most serious obstacle to progress in our health-care system. Being the most profit-oriented segment, it will therefore be the hardest to change. As difficult as it is to defend this industry, part of its problem lies in the regulatory structure for drug approval and the bloated $359 million it costs to develop and market drugs. These enormous expenses drive prices into the stratosphere and foster greed.

The most frightening aspect of the pharmaceutical industry, however, is its relationships with the nation's health-care providers, our medical doctors and the FDA. Within the hundreds of millions of dollars behind each drug lie regulatory jobs at the FDA and a $5,000 promotional allowance for the nation's 479,000 doctors.[13] In an exposé published in *Time* magazine some of these benefits to physicians were detailed. Wyeth Ayerst, for example, has offered to doctors 1,000 points toward American Airlines travel for each patient put on the hypertension drug Inderal, and Ciba-Geigy has given free Caribbean vacations to physicians for simply attending lectures on Estraderm.[24]

> The Task Force (FDA) considered many issues
> in its deliberations including to insure that the existence
> of dietary supplements (vitamins, minerals, amino acids,
> herbs and other) on the market does not act as a
> disincentive for drug development.
> *FDA TASK FORCE REPORT 1993* [25]

THE SOLUTION:

The only way change will occur in this industry is through consumer awareness and diligence on the part of medical ethicists. Government should offer incentives for drug companies to develop less expensive, safer and more natural medications while still allowing free enterprise to smaller purveyors of traditional medicines. This is certainly a Sisyphean task in itself.

The Food Industry

Among life's great dichotomies: Kids like junk food,
but their parents want them to eat right. The folks behind
the food are betting the kids win out . . . Companies are
appealing to a fertile audience: Children ages six to fourteen spend $7.3 billion a year and influence family buying
of more than $120 billion a year.

SELINA GUBER, PRESIDENT,
CHILDREN'S MARKET RESEARCH INC.[26]

THE PROBLEM:

How will we ever be healthy if our food is laden with
chemicals and depleted of its life-giving values? The
problem with the food industry is epitomized in the
above statement by Selina Guber.

THE SOLUTION:

The food industry is driven by market forces. Increased
pressure by consumer groups should continue to force
product development of healthier food choices.

The Medical Establishment

We've developed a medical system of specialists, who do
ordinary things at very special prices.

C. EVERETT KOOP, M.D.,
FORMER U.S. SURGEON GENERAL[27]

THE PROBLEM:

One of the most serious problems with the medical
profession is highlighted in the following combination
of facts:
1) Six of the ten leading causes of death among Americans are diet related, including heart disease, cancer,
stroke, diabetes mellitus, chronic liver disease and
atherosclerosis;
2) Data from the Association of the American Medical
Colleges concludes that in 1992, only one-fourth of the
127 medical schools in the United States taught nutrition
as a required course. The number of medical schools with
a required course in nutrition has actually decreased in
recent years.[28]

Besides poor priorities, established from the very beginning of the medical education process, physicians face serious ethical issues which might derail a positive change in the health-care system. A recent report in *JAMA* highlighted this when it concluded that "requests by physicians that drugs be added to a hospital formulary were strongly and specifically associated with the physicians' interactions with the companies manufacturing the drugs."[29] Also, what kind of ethical message is its representative body, the American Medical Association (AMA), sending to its constituents when a recent *New England Journal of Medicine* study concluded that the association financially supports the very positions it is supposedly working against (i.e., tobacco exports and lack of hand-gun legislation). The AMA actually gives more money to congressional members who oppose AMA positions on public-health issues than to those who support AMA positions.[30]

THE SOLUTION:

How can our health-care providers truly help us if they can never really understand the problem? A drastic and immediate change should be called for in the basic structure of medical education in the United States compelling it to include extensive courses in both holism and the ethics of healing. Last, a proposal that is inconceivable but worth mentioning: It is well known that in certain Asian cultures, healers have only been paid if their patients were kept healthy. Who would doubt that if we could make such a visionary shift in remuneration structure here that focus on details like nutrition would be adopted overnight.

The Insurance Industry

The insurance industry has driven the nation to the brink of bankruptcy. It is time for all Americans to stand up and say to the insurance industry: Enough is enough. We want our health-care system back.

HILLARY RODHAM CLINTON[31]

THE PROBLEM:

Premiums for health insurance are like a spider's web directly tied into the escalating costs of medical technology. Not only can fewer and fewer Americans afford health insurance but even those with insurance find that when it is finally needed for a catastrophic illness, their coverage has been dropped through a loophole or technicality. Instead of dealing with the roots of why so many of us are sick, a large segment of the insurance industry has chosen simply to adapt by raising premiums and dropping coverage. Sadly, the industry actually denies reimbursement for lower-cost alternative health-care treatments that are currently defined as experimental.

THE SOLUTION:

Insurance companies started on the right track when they reduced premiums for nonsmokers. What about people who eat a whole-food diet, exercise, practice stress reduction or take dietary supplements? Also, why should a drug treatment for arthritis be reimbursed at $100 while a $10 alternative ginger treatment be disallowed? The insurance companies could at least offer the choice. A few companies like American Western Life Insurance and Mutual of Omaha are proving that it can be done.♦

Ginger Accepts the Challenge

When the minds of the people are closed and wisdom is locked out, they remain tied to disease.

HUANG-TI, 2696-2598 B.C. (FROM THE NEI CHING SU WEN, OLDEST MEDICAL BOOK EXTANT) [32]

♦ American Western Life Insurance employs a team of naturopathic physicians and offers compensation for alternative treatments. Mutual of Omaha has recently decided to cover the *Reversal Program* as developed by Dean Ornish, M.D..

❦NOTE❧

There have been many people throughout time who have believed that plants possess a spirit. If we even briefly embrace this model, then it appears that ginger's credentials for flavor, safety, and historic and modern applications place it prominently among the promising and willing solutions to our current care crises.

───────────────

One of the principal reasons I have chosen to write about ginger, besides my personal attraction to the spice and its considerable health offerings, is ginger's potential as a catalyst for positive change. In an almost chilling reincarnation of its historical significance, ginger might again be in the center of a cataclysmic play.

Ginger by its very existence could safely, inexpensively and successfully challenge the foundations of some of the giants of the pharmaceutical industry and many of their flagship products totaling literally billions of dollars in annual sales.

Even more importantly, ginger might act as a representative of a limitless inventory of life-saving medicines. If spices like ginger can offer so many medical benefits, just imagine what other treasures might be waiting in the yet unexplored 99 percent of the world's flora. Considering that 25 percent of modern drugs are currently being synthesized or isolated from less than 1 percent of the world's flora, it is easy to understand why noted pharmacogonists like Dr. Norman Farnsworth have declared that there is a botanical treatment for every disease that faces humankind.

In our common spice ginger, we hold the promise of awakening our awareness to the vast potential herbs and natural healing modalities possess, a potential that can quite literally save our lives.

> For every disease that afflicts mankind, there is a treatment or a cure occurring naturally on this earth.
> DR. NORMAN FARNSWORTH, PHARMACOGINIST[33]

9

THE ESSENCE OF GINGER

☙❦❧☙

1. Ginger offers a variety of therapeutic effects which no modern drug can rival. Unfortunately, due to a monopolistic health-care system and a historically biased regulatory environment, full awareness of ginger's value has been limited.

2. Ginger is the most popular of hundreds of members of the Zingiberaceae family. To be botanically correct, ginger is a rhizome and not a root. It is available in many varieties, from mild to spicy, and requires tropical conditions and fertile soil for optimal growth.

3. Over a period of 5,000 years, ginger traveled from Southeast Asia to the New World. Considered a treasure by some of the great figures of history, its ancient trade helped shape nations and insure its worldwide cultivation.

4. The observed effects of ginger are the result of the interactions of more than 400 constituents which can be broken down into four major classes: taste, fragrance, nutrients and synergists. While most of the therapeutic focus is on

the pungent taste compounds, called gingerols and shogaols, ginger's protein-digesting enzyme and antioxidant are also key elements.

5. In an attempt to simplify or elucidate the dynamic of ginger's healing properties, a model of principal action and observed effect is offered.

6. When a combination of ginger's individual constituents interact in a therapeutically defined fashion, the combined activity is referred to as a principal action. A principal action can manifest itself in many observed effects.

7. Observed effects like anti-inflammatory, antiparasitic, antimicrobial and digestive benefit can all result from one principal action–i.e., enzyme action. An observed effect, such as an anti-inflammatory one, can also have a variety of principal actions at its root: enzyme, eicosanoid balance and antioxidant.

8. The dynamics of eicosanoids represent a key to understanding the diversity of ginger's actions. Eicosanoids are physiologically active compounds that the body synthesizes from essential fatty acids. When these elements become imbalanced, a wide variety of disease conditions can evolve.

9. The pharmaceutical industry has attempted to modulate eicosanoids to treat a host of disease conditions but has essentially failed because of serious side effects.

10. Ginger naturally helps balance these vitally important eicosanoids without side effects.

11. Over millennia, millions of people have enjoyed the benefits of ginger. For spiritual upliftment, digestive comfort and strength, stimulation and relief from infirmity, ginger has been heralded as the herb of choice and has been included in most of traditional Eastern formulas. Ginger is quite aptly described in the traditional language of Sanskrit as *vishwabhesaj*, the universal medicine.

12. In more recent times, in the early part of the twentieth century, more than 25,000 U.S. physicians, the Eclectics, lauded the pain-relieving and cold-fighting values of ginger.

13. Ginger was used historically in different regions of the world for the same basic therapeutic applications. These

include: analgesic, antiarthritic, wound healing, anthelmintic, antiulcer, stimulant and aphrodisiac properties, plus treatment of a variety of respiratory, reproductive and digestive complaints.

14. Intriguing studies by Danish researcher Srivastava and others illustrate ginger's therapeutic potential against arthritis. Ginger as a treatment offers many advantages over currently popular nonsteroidal anti-inflammatory drugs. Over a period of three to six months, clinical trials suggest that ginger is more effective than these commonly prescribed drugs and without serious side effects.

15. Ginger is a preventive treatment for critical cardiovascular disorders. Like aspirin, it holds the potential to prevent thousands of deaths from heart attacks and strokes as well as colon cancer. But unlike aspirin, it will have no side effects.

16. Ginger is a potentially powerful antiulcer treatment rivaling three of the nation's most popular drugs which account for $2.8 billion in sales annually.

17. The antiulcer effect of ginger is complemented by a host of other important digestive values which include relief of both diarrhea and constipation, liver protection and probiotic support.

18. The antinausea effect of ginger is well documented. From nausea resulting from chemotherapy and ocean travel to pregnancy and gynecological surgery, ginger is the natural treatment of choice.

19. Ginger, the bioavailability herb, assists the digestion of other nutrients and is a recommended addition to natural supplement regimes.

20. Parasites pose a much greater threat to the industrialized world than is generally recognized. Ginger exhibits a wide range of antiparasitic activities.

21. The historic observation that ginger is a cold remedy is a result of a combination of principal actions including eicosanoid balance, probiotic support, antitoxic and cytoprotective influences.

22. Ginger possesses a significant antimutagenic potential against such powerful carcinogens as benzo(a)pyrene and

the most toxic burned byproducts of the amino acid tryptophan. Research also warrants further investigation into ginger's anticancer properties and its role in a cancer-treatment program.

23. Ginger has been shown to affect positively parameters of health such as cholesterol and blood sugar and balance numerous body systems including the circulatory, respiratory and reproductive systems. Ginger's beneficial effects have also been demonstrated in external treatments with dramatic results.

24. Ginger is a remarkably safe herb. No modern pharmaceutical can compete with its range of therapeutic properties and absence of adverse side effects. Care and moderation should be exercised when using ginger during pregnancy and before surgery. Up to 1 gram daily of the powdered herb should be a safe preventive dosage for the general population. In all cases, introduction of ginger into the diet should be gradual.

25. The effectiveness of ginger will be dependent upon the quality of the rhizome. Since commercial ginger is subject to many potential levels of chemical contamination, organically certified products are recommended.

26. Both fresh and dry ginger are recommended forms for supplementation. There will be different properties gained from each. Ginger is commercially available in many forms including fresh, dried, syrup, capsules and extract.

27. With a health-care system that is widely recognized in crisis and in danger of bankrupting this country, natural and traditional remedies offer both a safe and economical potential to save lives and drastically improve the nation's health.

28. Government and the pharmaceutical, food, medical and insurance industries have much at stake in the current system's continuation. Whether or not the public will ever realize the full daily tonic and healing value of ginger as well as the huge potential of countless other traditional remedies will be dependent upon the political strength of the growing alternative- and self-health-care movements.

Glossary

🙘🙚🙘🙚

Abortifacient – An agent that produces abortion.

Adaptogenic – Used to describe an herb or natural substance that acts in a nonspecific manner to promote an advantageous change in metabolic functioning.

Aggregating – Uniting together in a cluster.

Analeptic – A restorative remedy; a central nervous system stimulant.

Analgesic – A condition in which stimuli are perceived but are not interpreted as pain; usually accompanied by sedation without loss of consciousness.

Angina pectoris – Severe constricting pain in the chest, often radiating from the pericardium to the left shoulder and down the arm, due to obstruction of blood supply to the heart muscle usually caused by coronary disease.

Anthelmintic – An agent that destroys or expels intestinal worms.

Antibacterial – Destructive to or preventing the growth of bacteria.

Anticathartic – An agent that inhibits purging or evacuating of the bowels.

Antidiabetic – Preventing or inhibiting the development of diabetes (any of several carbohydrate metabolic disorders marked by excessive discharge of urine and persistent thirst).

Antiemetic – A remedy that tends to control nausea and vomiting.

Antifungal – Inhibiting the growth of fungi, any of numerous plants lacking chlorophyll and including yeasts, molds, smuts and mushrooms.

Anti-inflammatory – Reducing inflammation by acting on body mechanisms, without directly antagonizing the causative agent; denoting agents such as antihistamines and glucocorticoids.

Antimetastatic – Preventing the shifting of a disease (usually referring to cancer) from one part of the body to another part.

The *Stedman's Medical Dictionary* (25th edition) is the source for this glossary.

Antimutagenic – Inhibiting the ability to cause cell mutations and the potential of cancer.

Antioxidant – An agent that inhibits oxidation and thus prevents rancidity of oils or fats or the deterioration of other materials through oxidative processes.

Antipyretic – An agent that reduces fever.

Antithrombic – Inhibiting or preventing the effects of thrombin (an enzyme in blood that facilitates blood clotting) in such a manner that blood does not coagulate.

Antitumor – Inhibiting the development of tumors or swellings in the body.

Antitussive – A cough remedy or reliever.

Antiulcer – Inhibiting the development of ulcers or lesions on the surface of the skin or a mucous surface, caused by superficial loss of tissue, usually from inflammation.

Antiviral – Inhibiting the development of a virus, any of various submicroscopic pathogens consisting essentially of a core of a single nucleic acid surrounded by a protein coat, having the ability to replicate only inside a living cell.

Aphrodisiac – Anything that arouses or increases sexual desire.

Arrhythmia – Loss of rhythm, denoting especially irregularity of the heartbeat.

Arteriosclerosis – Hardening of the arteries.

Ascites – Accumulation of fluid in the abdomen.

Bioavailability – The physiological availability of a given amount of a drug, as distinct from its chemical potency.

Cardiotonic – Exerting a favorable effect upon the action of the heart.

Carminative – Preventing the formation or causing the expulsion of gas; an agent that relieves flatulence.

Cholagogic – An agent that promotes bile flow into the intestine, especially as a result of gall bladder contraction.

Colitis – Inflammation of the colon.

Corticosteroids – Steroid produced by the adrenal cortex.

Cyclooxygenase – The enzyme principally responsible for the production of prostaglandin endoperoxides and subsequent prostaglandins and thromboxanes.

Cytotoxic – Detrimental or destructive to cells.

Diaphoretic – An agent that increases perspiration.

Dimenhydrinate – An amine salt used for motion sickness.

Dyskenisia – Difficulty in performing voluntary movements.

Edema – Accumulation of excessive amounts of watery fluid in cells and tissues.

Eicosanoids – The physiologically active substances derived from arachidonic acid, i.e., the prostaglandins, leukotrienes, and thromboxanes.

Also known as the arachidonic acid cascade.

Emesis – Vomiting.

Emmenagogue – An agent that induces or increases menstrual flow.

Enzyme – Organic catalyst; a protein, secreted by cells, that acts as a catalyst to induce chemical changes in other substances, itself remaining apparently unchanged by the process.

Expectorant – An agent promoting secretion from the mucous membrane of the air passages or facilitating its expulsion.

Febrifuge – An agent that reduces fever.

Filariasis – The presence of filariae or nematodes in the tissues of the body, or in blood or tissue fluids.

Fumigant – Any vaporous substance used as a disinfectant or pesticide.

Fungicide – Any substance that has a destructive killing action upon fungi.

Galactagogue – An agent that promotes the secretion and flow of milk.

Hepatotoxic – Relating to an agent that damages the liver, or pertaining to any such action.

Hypocholesteremic – Denoting the presence of abnormally small amounts of cholesterol in the circulating blood.

Hypoglycemia – An abnormally small concentration of glucose in the circulating blood, i.e., less than the minimum of the normal range.

Immune supportive – Aiding in the resistance to an infectious disease; helping to free from the possibility of acquiring a given infectious disease.

Ischemic – Relating to or affected by ischemia, the local anemia due to mechanical obstruction (mainly arterial narrowing) of the blood supply.

Leukotrienes – Products of arachidonic acid metabolism with postulated physiologic activity such as mediators of inflammation and roles in allergic reactions; differ from the related prostaglandins and thromboxanes by not having a central ring.

Motility – The power of spontaneous movement.

Mucolytic – Capable of dissolving, digesting, or liquefying mucus.

Mutagenic – Having the power to cause cell mutations and the potential for cancer.

Myelopoiesis – Formation of the tissue elements of bone marrow, or any of the types of blood cells derived from bone marrow, or both processes.

Nematode – A common name for any roundworm of the phylum Nematoda.

Necrotizing – Causing the pathologic death of one or more cells.

Neutrophil – A mature white blood cell formed in the bone marrow and released into the circulating blood where they normally represent 54 to 65 percent of the total number of white blood cells.

Osteoarthritis – Degenerative joint disease; arthritis characterized by erosion of joint cartilage, either primary or secondary to trauma or other conditions, which becomes soft, frayed, and thinned; pain and loss of function result.

Panacea – A cure-all; a remedy claimed to be a curative for all diseases.

Parturition – The act of giving birth; childbirth.

Pathogen – Any agent that causes diseases.

Phagocytosis – The process of the immune system in which ingestion and digestion by cells of solid substances, e.g., other cells, bacteria, bits of dead tissue, foreign particles, occurs.

Placebo – An inert compound identical in appearance to material being tested in experimental research, which may or may not be known to the physician and/or patient, administered to distinguish between drug action and suggestive effect of the material under study.

Platelet aggregation – A crowded mass or cluster of blood platelets.

Preeclampsia – Development of hypertension with excess protein in the urine or edema, or both, due to pregnancy or the influence of a recent pregnancy; it occurs after the twentieth week of gestation but may develop before this time.

Probiotic support – Fostering symbiosis, the association of two organisms that enhances the life processes of both. Often used to describe dietary supplements that encourage a healthy microbial environment.

Prostaglandin – Any of a class of physiologically active substances present in many tissues, with effects such as vasodilation, vasoconstriction, stimulation of intestinal or bronchial smooth muscle, uterine stimulation, and antagonism to hormones influencing lipid metabolism.

Rheumatoid arthritis – Systemic disease that affects connective tissue involving many joints accompanied by thickening of articular soft tissues which become eroded. Often chronic and progressive leading to disability.

Rhizome – Creeping, underground stem of a plant.

Rubefacient – Causing a reddening of the skin.

Schistosomiasis – A chronic and often debilitating infection with a species of Schistosoma, a genus of trematodes, including the blood flukes of man and domestic animals.

Sciatica – Pain in the lower back and hip radiating down the back of the thigh into the leg, usually due to a herniated lumbar disk.

Serotonin – A vasoconstrictor, liberated by the blood platelets, that inhibits gastric secretion and stimulates smooth muscle.

Sialogogue – An agent promoting the flow of saliva.

Synergist – A structure, agent, or physiologic process that aids the action of another.

Synthetase – An enzyme catalyzing the synthesis–or composition–of a specific substance.

Systemic – Relating to a system, the entire organism.

Thermoregulatory – Controlling temperature.

Thromboxanes – A group of compounds, included in the eicosanoids, biochemically related to the prostaglandins and formed from them through a series of steps involving the formation of an endoperoxide by a cyclooxygenase. Thromboxanes are so named from their influence on platelet aggregation and the formation of the oxygen-containing six-membered ring.

Thrombosis – Clotting within a blood vessel which may cause infarction–or sudden insufficiency of blood supply–of tissues supplied by the vessel.

Trematode – Common name for a fluke of the class Trematoda, flatworms with leaf-shaped bodies and two muscular suckers.

Ulcer – A lesion on the surface of the skin or mucous surface caused by superficial loss of tissue, usually with inflammation.

Ulcerogenic – Ulcer producing.

Vasoconstriction – Narrowing of the blood vessels.

Vasospasm – Contraction or extreme tension of the muscular coats of the blood vessels.

GINGER'S CONSTITUENTS
AND ACTIONS

An herb is an infinitely complex array of elements. To create an observed therapeutic effect, each of these hundreds of elements interacts with the others in a cascade that defies explanation. This section is included to give the reader a sense of just how miraculous a plant's activities are and how presumptuous it is to think that one can isolate the "active" element from a plant.

Although there are serious limitations to active constituent isolation, this partial breakdown on ginger constituents reveals an awe-inspiring array of elements. Many of these compounds have collectively been the subject of thousands of studies. Besides the constituents already mentioned, of particular note here are ascorbic acid, caffeic acid, capsaicin, beta-sitosterol, beta-carotene, curcumin, kaempferol, lecithin, limonene, quercetin, selenium and tryptophan.

This section combines the monumental works of botanist James Duke of the United States Department of Agriculture,◆ and Norman Farnsworth, Research Professor at the University of Illinois.[1-4]

◆ Professor Duke's *Handbook of Biologically Active Phytochemicals and Their Activities* is the principal source for the listed biological activities.

1. ACETALADEHYDE: fungicide respiroparalytic

2. 2-HEPTYL ACETATE

3. 2-NONYL ACETATE

4. ALPHA-FENCHYL ACETATE

5. ACETIC-ACID: antiotitic, antivaginitic, bactericide, expectorant, fungicide, mucolytic, osteolytic, protisticide, spermicide, ulcerogenic, verrucolytic

6. ACETONE: CNS-depressant, narcotic

7. ALANINE: Cancer preventive

8. ALBUMIN

9. ALLO-AROMADENDRENE

10. ALLO-AROMADENDRINE

11. ALUMINUM: Antivaginitic, candidicide, encephalopathic

12. GAMMA-AMINOBUTYRIC-ACID: analeptic, antihypertensive, antilethargic, diuretic, neurotransmitter

13. ALPHA-AMORPHENE

14. GAMMA-AMORPHENE

15. ANGELICOIDENOL-2-0- BETA-D-GLUCOPYRANOSIDE

16. ARGININE: antiencephalopathic, antihepatitic, anti-infertility, diuretic

17. AROMADENDRENE

18. AROMADENDRIN: cancer-preventive

19. ASCORBIC-ACID: antiChron's, anticold, antidecubitic, antidote (paraquat), antiedemic, antilepric, antimigraine, antinitrosic, antioxidant, antiscorbutic, antiseptic, cancer preventive, detoxicant, diuretic, hypotensive, mucolytic, urinary acidulant, vulnerary

20. ASH

21. ASPARAGINE: antisickling, diuretic

22. ASPARTIC-ACID: antimorphinic, neuroexcitant

23. BENZALDEHYDE: anesthetic, antipeptic, antiseptic, antispasmodic, antitumor, insectifuge, narcotic

24. 3-PHENYL BENZALDEHYDE

25. 4-PHENYL BENZALDEHYDE

26. ALPHA-BERGAMOTENE

27. TRANS-ALPHA-BERGAMOTENE

28. BISABOLENE

29. ALPHA-BISABOLENE

30. BETA-BISABOLENE

31. CIS-GAMMA-BISABOLENE

32. BETA-BISABOLOL

33. BORNEOL: analgesic, anti-inflammatory, febrifuge, hepatoprotectant, berbicide, insectifuge, spasmolytic

34. D-BORNEOL

35. BORNEOL ACETATE

36. (+)-BORNEOL

37. ISO-BORNEOL

38. BORNYL-ACETATE: antifeedant, bactericide, insectifuge, viricide

39. BORON: androgenic, antiosteoporotic, estrogenic

40. BETA-BOURBONENE

41. BUTANAL

42. 2-MENTHYLBUTANAL

43. 2-METHYLBUTANAL

44. 3-METHYLBUTANAL

45. 2-BUTANOL

46. SEC-BUTANOL

47. TERT-BUTANOL

48. 2-METHYL-BUT-3-EN-2-OL

49. N-BUTYRALDEHYDE

50. ALPHA-CADINENE

51. DELTA-CADINENE

52. GAMMA-CADINENE

53. ALPHA-CADINOL

54. 10-ALPHA-CADINOL

55. CAFFEIC-ACID: antiflu, antihepatotoxic, antiherpetic, antioxidant, antiseptic, antispasmodic, antitumor, antitumor promoter, antiviral, bactericide, cancer preventive, choleretic, fungicide, hepatoprotective, hepatotropic, histamine inhibitor, leukotriene inhibitor, lipoxygenase inhibitor, tumorigenic, viricide, vulnerary

56. CALAMENENE

57. CALCIUM

58. CAMPHENE: insectifuge

59. CAMPHENE-HYDRATE

60. CYCLOCOPACAMPHENE

61. CAMPHOR: allelopathic, analgesic, anesthetic, antifeedant, antifibrositic, antineuralgic, antipruritic, antiseptic, cancer-preventive, carminative, CNS-stimulant, convulsant, counterirritant, deliriant, ecbolic, emetic, expectorant, herbicide, insectifuge, respiroinhibitor, rubefacient, stimulant

62. CAPRIC-ACID: fungicide

63. CAPRYLIC-ACID: candidicide, fungicide

64. CAPSAICIN: analgesic, anesthetic, antiaggregant, anti-inflammatory, antineuralgic, antinociceptive, antioxidant, antiulcer, cancer preventive, carcinogenic, cardiotonic, cyclooxygenase inhibitor, diaphoretic, hypothermic, irritant, 5-lipoxygenase inhibitor, neurotoxic, repellent, respirosensitizer, sialogogue

65. CARBOHYDRATES

66. CAR-3-ENE

67. DELTA-3-CARENE: bactericide, anti-inflammatory, insectifuge

68. CARVOTANACETONE

69. BETA-CAROTENE: antiacne, antiaging, anticoronary, antilupus,

antiozenic, antiphotophobic, antiPMS, antiporphyric, antitumor, antiulcer, cancer preventive, immunostimulant

70. CARYOPHYLLENE: antiedemic, anti-inflammatory, insectifuge, perfumery, spasmolytic, termitifuge

71. CARYOPHYLLENE OXIDE: antiedemic, anti-inflammatory

72. BETA-CARYOPHYLLENE

73. CEDOROL

74. CHAVICOL: fungicide, nematicide

75. CHLOROGENIC-ACID: allergenic, antifeedant, antihepatotoxic, antioxidant, antipolio, antiseptic, antitumor promoter, antiviral, bactericide, cancer preventive, choleretic, clastogenic, diuretic, histamine inhibitor, juvabional, leukotriene inhibitor, lipoxygenase inhibitor

76. CHROMIUM: Insulinogenic

77. CINEOL

78. 1,4-CINEOLE

79. 1,8-CINEOLE: allelopathic, anesthetic, antibronchitic, anticatarrh, antilaryngitic, antipharyngitic, antirhinitic, antiseptic, antitussive, bactericide, choleretic, CNS stimulant, counterirritant, dentifrice, expectorant, fungicide, hepatotonic, herbicide, hypotensive, insectifuge, rubefacient, sedative

80. 2-HYDROXY-1,8-CINEOL

81. CITRAL: antihistaminic, antiseptic, bactericide, cancer preventive, fungicide, herbicide, perfumery, sedative, teratogenic

82. CITRONELLAL: antiseptic, bactericide, embryotoxic, insectifuge, perfumery, sedative, tertogenic

83. CITRONELLOL: bactericide, candidicide, fungicide, herbicide, perfumery, sedative

84. CITRONELLYL-ACETATE

85. COBALT

86. CUBEBOL

87. CUMINYL ALCOHOL

88. DOCOSANE

89. EICOSANE

90. HENICOSANE

91. TRICOSANE

92. COPAENE

93. ALPHA-COPAENE

94. COPPER: contraceptive

95. P-COUMARIC-ACID: antineoplastic, bactericide, cancer preventive, choleretic, lipoxygenase inhibitor, prostaglandin-synthesis inhibitor

96. CRYPTONE

97. CUMENE: narcotic

98. CUPARENE

99. ALPHA-CURCUMENE: antitumor, anti-inflammatory

100. (+)-ALPHA-CURCUMENE

101. AR-CURCUMENE

102. BETA-CURCUMENE

103. CURCUMIN: antiaggregant, anticholecystitic, antiedemic, anti-inflammatory, antilymphomic, antimutagenic, antiprostaglandin, antitumor, antitumor promoter, bactericide, cancer preventive, cardiodepressant, cholagogue, choleretic, cyclooxygenase inhibitor, cytotoxic, dye, fungicide, hepatoprotective, hypotensive, 5-lipoxygenase inhibitor, spasmolytic

104. HEXAHYDROCURCUMIN: choleretic, cholagogue

105. DEMETHYL-HEXAHYDRO-CURCUMIN

106. CYCLOSATIVENE

107. P-CYMENE: analgesic, antiflu, antirheumatalgic, bactericide, fungicide, herbicide, insectifuge, viricide

108. P-CYMEN-8-OL

109. CYSTEINE: antiaddisonian, anticytotoxic, antiophthalmic, antioxidant, antitumor, antiulcer, cancer preventive, detoxicant

110. CYSTINE: adjuvant, antihomocystinuric

111. DECANAL

112. N-DECANAL

113. UNDECANAL

114. DODECANE

115. HEPTADECANE

116. HEXADECANE

117. NONADECANE

118. OCTADECANE

119. PENTADECANE

120. TETRADECANE

121. TRIDECANE

122. UNDECANE

123. 3-6-EPOXY-1-(4-HYDROXY-3- METHOXY-PHENYL) DECA-3-5-DIENE

124. 3(R)-5(S)-DIACETOXY-1-(3-4-DI-METHOXY-PHENYL) DECANE

125. 3(R)-5(S)-DIACETOXY-1-(4- HYDROXY-3-METHOXY-PHENYL) DECANE

126. 3(R)-ACETOXY-5(S)-HYDROXY- 1-(4-HYDROXY-3-METHOXY-PHENYL) DECANE

127. 5(S)-3(R)-DIHYDROXY-1-(4- HYDROXY-3-METHOXY-PHENYL) DECANE

128. 5(S)-ACETOXY-3(R)-HYDROXY- 1-(4-HYDROXY-3-METHOXY-PHENYL) DECANE

129. DECYLALDEHYDE

130. 6-DEHYDROGINGERDIONE: prostaglandin suppressor

131. 6,10-DEHYDROGINGERDIONE

132. 10-DEHYDROGINGERDIONE: anticholeretic, prostaglandin suppressor

133. 6-DIHYDROGINGERDIONE

134. DELPHINIDIN: allelochemic, cancer preventive

135. DIETHYL-SULFIDE

136. DODECANOIC-ACID

137. BETA-ELEMENE

138. ELEMOL

139. BETA-ELEMENE

140. DELTA-ELEMENE

141. GAMMA-ELEMENE

142. ELEMOL

143. ESSENTIAL OIL

144. 10-EPIZONARENE

145. 8-BETA-17-EPOXY-LABD- TRANS-12-ENE-15,16-DIAL

146. ETHYL-ACETATE: antispasmodic, carminative, CNS depressant, stimulant

147. ETHYL-MYRISTATE

148. ALPHA-EUDESMOL

149. BETA-EUDESMOL: antianoxic, antipeptic, CNS inhibitor, hepatoprotective

150. GAMMA-EUDESMOL

151. METHYL-ETHER-ISO-EUGENOL

152. FARNESAL: juvabional

153. FARNESENE

154. ALPHA-FARNESENE

155. TRANS-ALPHA-FARNESENE

156. BETA-FARNESENE

157. TRANS-BETA-FARNESENE: pheromone

158. FARNESOL: juvabional, perfumery

159. FAT

160. FERULIC-ACID: allelopathic, analgesic, antiaggregant, antidysmenor-rheic, antispasmodic, antitumor, antitumor promoter, antiviral, arteriodilator, bactericide, cancer preventive, cardiac, choleretic, fungicide, hepatotropic, preservative, uterosedative

161. FIBER: antitumor, antidiabetic, antiobesity, cancer preventive, cardioprotective, hypocholesteremic, hypotensive, laxative

162. FLUORIDE

163. FLUORINE

164. FRUCTOSE: antiketotic, neoplastic

165. FURANOGERMENONE

166. FURFURAL: antiseptic, fungicide, insecticide

167. GADOLEIC-ACID

168. GALANOLACTONE: anti-5HT3 activity

169. GERANIAL: bactericide

170. CIS-GERANIC-ACID

171. TRANS-GERANIC-ACID

172. GERANIOL: antiseptic, cancer preventive, candidicide, embryotoxic, fungicide, insectifuge, insectiphile, perfumery, sedative

173. GERANIOL ACETATE

174. GERANYL-ACETATE

175. GERMACRENE B

176. GERMACRENE D: pheromonal

177. GERMANIUM

178. GINGEDIACETATE

179. 4-GINGEDIACETATE

180. 6-GINGEDIACETATE

181. 4-GINGEDIOL

182. 6-GINGEDIOL

183. 6-GINGEDIOL-ACETATE

184. 6-GINGEDIOL-ACETATE- METHYL-ETHER

185. 6-GINGEDIOL-DIACETATE

186. 6-GINGEDIOL-DIACETATE- METYYL-ETHER

187. 6-GINGEDIOL-METHYL- ETHER

188. 8-GINGEDIOL

189. 10-GINGEDIOL

190. 4-GINGERDIONE

191. 6-GINGERDIONE: prostaglandin suppressor

192. 8-GINGERDIONE

193. 10-GINGERDIONE: prostaglandin suppressor

194. 6-10-GINGERDIONE

195. GINGERENONE-A: anticoccidioid, fungicide

196. GINGERENONE-B: fungicide

197. GINGERENONE-C: fungicide

198. GINGERGLYCOLIPID-A

199. GINGERGLYCOLIPID-B

200. GINGERGLYCOLIPID-C

201. GINGEROL: cancer preventive, hepatoprotective, molluscicide

202. 3-GINGEROL

203. 4-GINGEROL

204. 5-GINGEROL

205. 6-GINGEROL: analgesic, anti-5-HT, antiemetic, antipyretic, antitussive, cardiotonic, cholagogue, depressor, hepatoprotective, hypotensive, prostaglandin suppressor, sedative

206. (+)-6-GINGEROL

207. (S)(+)-6-GINGEROL

208. 6-GINGEROL-METHYL

209. 7-GINGEROL

210. 8-GINGEROL: anti-5-HT, cardiotonic, enteromotility enhancer

211. 8-GINGEROL-METHYL

9-GINGEROL

212. 10-GINGEROL: cardiotonic

213. 10-GINGEROL-METHYL

214. 12-GINGEROL

215. 12-GINGEROL-METHYL

216. 14-GINGEROL

217. 16-GINGEROL

218. DIHYDRO-GINGEROL

219. GINGEROL-METHYL

220. GINGEROL-METHYL-ETHER

221. GINGERONE

222. 6-GINGESULFONIC ACID

223. GLANOLACTONE-

224. GLANOLACTONE GLOBULIN

225. GLUCOSE: acetylcholinergic, antihepatotoxic, antiketotic, hyperglycemic, memory enhancer

226. GLUTAMIC-ACID: antalkali, antiepileptic, antihyperammonemic, antiretardation, anxiolytic

227. GLUTELIN

228. GLYCINE: antiacid, antidote, antiencephalopathic, antigastritic, antipruritic, antiulcer, cancer preventive

229. GLYOXAL

230. METHOXY GLYOXAL

231. GUAIOL: termitifuge

232. 6-METHYL-HEPT-5-EN-2-OL

233. 6-METHYL-HEPT-5-EN-2-ONE

234. HEPTAN-2-OL

235. HEPTAN-2-ONE

236. HEPTANE

237. N-HEPTANE

238. 2-2-4-TRIMETHYL-HEPTANE

239. 3(S)-5(S)-DIACETOXY-1-(4'- HYDROXY-3'-5'-DIMETHOXY-PHENYL)-7-(4"-HYDROXY-3"-METHOXY-PHENYL HEPTANE\

240. 3(S)-5(S)-DIHYDROXY-1-(4'- Hydroxy-3'-5'-DIMETHOXY-PHENYL)-7-(4"-HYDROXY-3"-METHOXY-PHENYL) HEPTANE

241. 3-5-DIACETOXY-1-(4- HYDROXY-3-5-DIMETHOXY-PHENYL)-7-(4-HYDROXY-3-METHOXY-PHENYL) HEPTANE

242. 3-5-DIACETOXY-1-7-BIS-(4- HYDROXY-3-METHOXY-PHENYL) MESO-HEPTANE

243. 1-7-BIS-(4-HYDROXY-3- METHOXY-PHENYL) HEPTANE- 3(S)-DIOL

244. METHYL-HEPTENONE

245. 2-HEPTANONE

246. HEXANAL

247. 2-HEXANONE

248. HEXAN-1-AL

249. HEXAN-1-OL

250. HEXANOL: antiseptic

251. CIS-HEXAN-3-OL

252. TRANS-2-HEXENAL

253. BETA-HIMACHALENE: anti-inflammatory, insecticide

254. HISTIDINE: antiarteriosclerotic, antiulcer

255. HUMULENE

256. P-HYDROXYBENZOIC-ACID: antisickling, bactericide, cancer preventive

257. 1-(4-HYDROXY-3-METHOXY PHENYL)-3,5-OCTANEDIOL

258. 1-(4-HYDROXY-3-METHOXY PHENYL)-3,5-DIACETOXYOCTANE

259. BETA-IONONE: cancer preventive

260. IRON: antiakathisic, antienemic

261. ISOEUGENOL-METHYL-ETHER

262. ISOGINGERENONE-B: fungicide

263. ISOLEUCINE: antiencephalopathic, antipellagric

264. ISOPUEGOL

265. ISOVALERALDEHYDE

266. JUNIPER CAMPHOR

267. KAEMPFEROL: antifertility, antihistaminic, anti-inflammatory, antioxidant, antispasmodic, antitumor promoter, antiulcer, cancer preventive, choleretic, diuretic, HIV-RT-inhibitor, hypotensive, mutagenic, natriuretic, spasmolytic, teratologic

268. KILOCALORIES

269. LAURIC-ACID

270. LECITHIN: antialzheimeran, antiataxic, anticirrhotic, antidementic, antidyskinetic, antieczemic, antimorphinistic, antioxidant (synergist), antipsoriac, antisclerodermic, antiseborrheic, antisprue, antiTourette's, cholinogenic, hepatoprotective, hypocholesterolemic, lipotropic

271. LEUCINE: antiencephalopathic

272. ISOLEUCINE

273. LIMONENE: achne inhibitor, anticancer, antilithic, bactericide, cancer preventive, herbicide, insectifuge, insecticide, irritant, sedative, viricide

274. LINALOOL: antiseptic, bactericide, cancer preventive, fungicide, insectifuge, perfumery, sedative, spasmolytic, termitifuge, tumor promoter, viricide

275. LINALOOL OXIDE

276. TRANS-LINALOOL-OXIDE

277. LINALYL ACETATE

278. LINOLEIC-ACID: antiarteriosclerotic, antifibrinolytic, antigranular, cancer preventive, hepatoprotective, insectifuge

279. ALPHA-LINOLENIC-ACID: cancer preventive

280. LYSINE: antialkalotic, hypoarginanemic

281. MAGNESIUM: hypotensive

282. MANGANESE: antianemic, antidyskinetic

283. 2-METHYL-BUT-3-EN-2-OL

284. CIS-P-MENTH-2-EN-1-OL

285. TRANS-P-MENTH-2-EN-1-OL

286. P-MENTHA-1-5-DIEN-7-OL

287. P-MENTHA-2-8-DIEN-1-OL

288. P-MENTHAL-1-5-DIEN-8-OL

289. MENTHOL-ACETATE

290. P-METHA-1-8-DIEN-7-OL

291. METHIONINE: antidote (acetominaphen, paracetamol), antieczemic, cancer preventive, emetic, glutathionigenic, hepatoprotective, lipotropic, urine acidifier, urine deodorant

292. METHYL-ACETATE

293. METHYL-CAPRYLATE

294. 6-METHYLGINGEDIACETATE

295. 6-METHYLGINGEDIOL

296. METHYL-GLYOXAL

297. METHYL-ISOBUTYL-KETONE

298. METHYL-NONYL-KETONE

299. METHYL-6-SHOGAOL

300. METHYL-8-SHOGAOL

301. METHYL-10-SHOGAOL

302. MUFA

303. ALPHA-MUUROLENE

304. GAMMA-MUUROLENE

305. MYRCENE: antinociceptive, bactericide, insectifuge, spasmolytic

306. BETA-MYRCENE: cancer preventive, perfumery

307. MYRICETIN: allelochemic, antifeedant, antigastric, anti-inflammatory, cancer preventive, diuretic, larvistat

308. MYRISTIC-ACID: cancer preventive, cosmetic

309. MYRTENAL

310. ALPHA-NEGINATENE

311. NEOISOPULEGOL

312. NERAL: bactericide

313. NEROL: bactericide, perfumery

314. NEROL OXIDE

315. NEROLIDOL

316. 9-OXO-NEROLIDOL

317. TRANS-NEROLIDOL

318. NIACIN: antiacrodynic, antiamplyopic, antianginal, antidysphagic, antineuralgic, antipellagric, antiscotomic, antivertigo, cancer preventive, hepatoprotective, hypoglycemic, vasodilator

319. NICKEL

320. NITROGEN

321. NONANAL

322. NONANE

323. N-NONANE

324. A-NONANONE

325. N-NONANONE

326. NONYL-ALDEHYDE

327. NONAN-2-OL

328. N-NONANOL

329. 2-NONANONE

330. CIS-OCIMENE

331. 2-6-DIMETHYL OCTA-2-6-DIENE-1-8-DIOL

332. 2-6-DIMETHYL OCTA-3-7-DIENE-1-6-DIOL

333. OCTANAL

334. 1-OCTANAL: fungicide, perfumery

335. OCTANE

336. N-OCTANE

337. 2-OCTANOL: perfumery

338. N-OCTANOL

339. TRANS-OCTEN-2-AL

340. OLEIC-ACID: anemiagenic, cancer preventive, choleretic, insectifuge, irritant, percutaneostimulant

341. OXALIC-ACID: antiseptic, fatal, hemostatic, renotoxic

342. 9-OXO-NEROLIDOL

343. PALMITIC-ACID: antifibrinolytic

344. PALMITOLEIC-ACID

345. PANTOTHENIC-ACID

346. PARADOL

347. 4-PARADOL

348. 6-PARADOL

349. PATCHOULI-ALCOHOL: antiplaque, bactericide, fungicide

350. PENTANAL

351. PENTAN-2-OL

352. 4-METHYL-2-PENTANONE

353. PENTOSANS

354. PERILLEN

355. PERILLENE

356. PHELLANDRAL

357. ALPHA-PHELLANDRENE: insectiphile

358. BETA-PHELLANDRENE: perfumery

359. (+)-BETA-PHELLANDRENE

360. PHENYLALANINE: anti–attention deficit disorder, antidepressant, antiparkinsonian, antisickling, antivitiligic, tremorigenic

361. PHOSPHATIDIC-ACID

362. PHOSPHORUS

363. PHYTOSTEROLS

364. ALPHA-PINENE: allelochemic, anti-inflammatory, cancer preventive, coleoptiphile, insectfuge, insectiphile

365. BETA-PINENE: insectifuge

366. PIPECOLIC-ACID

367. POTASSIUM

368. PROLAMINE

369. PROLINE

370. PROPANOL

371. N-PROPANOL

372. PROPIONALDEHYDE

373. PROTEIN

374. NEO-ISO-PULEGOLE

375. PUFA : antiacne, antieczemic, antiMS, antipolyneuritic

376. QUERCETIN: aldose-reductase inhibitor, allelochemic, antiaggregant, antiallergenic, antianaphylactic, anticataract, antidermatitic, antifeedant, anti-flu, antigastric, antihepatotoxic, antiherpetic, antihistaminic, antihydrophobic, anti-inflammatory, antileukotrienic, antilipoperoxidant, antioxidant, antiperme-ability, antiraducular, antispasmodic, antitumor, antiviral, bactericide, cancer preventive, capillariprotective, cytotoxic, HIV-RT inhibitor, juvabional, larvis-tat, lipoxygenase inhibitor, mast-cell stabilizer, mutagenic, spasmolytic, terato-logic, tumorigenic, vasodilator, xanthine-oxidase inhibitor

377. RAFFINOSE

378. RIBOFLAVIN: antiarabiflavinotic, anticheilotic, antidecubitic, antiker-atitic, antimigraine, antipellagric, antiphotophobic, cancer preventive

379. ROSEFURAN

380. SABINENE

381. CIS-SABINENE HYDRATE

382. SELENIUM: anorexic, antidote (mercury), antikeshan, antiosteoarthritic, antioxidant, antiulcerogenic, cancer preventive, depressant, prostaglandin sparer

383. CIS-SELINEN-4-OL

384. ALPHA-SELINENE

385. BETA-SELINENE

386. GAMMA-SELINENE

387. SELINA-4, 11-DIENE

388. SELINA-3, 11-DIENE

389. SELINA-3(7), 11-DIENE

390. SERINE: cancer preventive

391. CIS-SESQUISABINENE-HYDRATE

392. SESQUIPHELLANDRENE

393. BETA-SESQUIPHELLAN DRENE

394. BETA-SESQUIPHELLANDROL

395. CIS-BETA-SESQUIPHELLAN DROL

396. TRANS-BETA-SESQUIPHEL-LANDROL

397. CIS-SESQUISABINENE-HYDRATE

398. SESQUITERPENE ALCOHOL

399. SESQUITERPENE HYDROCARBON

400. SFA

401. SHIKIMIC-ACID: bruchifuge, carcinogenic, ileorelaxant, mutagenic

402. SHOGAOL: anti-inflammatory, cyclooxygenase-inhibitor, hypotensive, 5-lipoxygenase inhibitor, molluscicide

403. 4-SHOGAOL

404. 6-SHOGAOL: analgesic, anti-5-HT, antipyretic, antitussive, CNS depressant, enteromotility enhancer, hepatoprotective, hypotensive, prostaglandin suppressor, sedative, sympathomimetic, vasoconstrictor

405. CIS-6-SHOGAOL

406. 6-METHYL-SHOGAOL

407. ANTI-METHYL-6-SHOGAOL

408. SYN-METHYL-6-SHOGAOL

409. TRAN-6-SHOGOAL

410. 8-SHOGAOL

411. CIS-8-SHOGAOL

412. 8-METHYL-SHOGAOL

413. ANTI-METHYL-8-SHOGAOL

414. SYN-METHYL-8-SHOGAOL

415. TRAN-8-SHOGAOL

416. 10-SHOGAOL

417. CIS-10-SHOGAOL

418. ANTI-METHYL-10-SHOGAOL

419. SYN-METHYL-10-SHOGAOL

420. TRANS-10-SHOGAOL

421. CIS-12-SHOGAOL

422. TRANS-12-SHOGAOL

423. SILICON

424. BETA-SITOSTEROL: androgenic, anorexic, antiadenomic, antiandrogenic, antiestrogenic, antifeedant, antifertility, antigonadotrophic, anti-inflammatory, antileukemic, antimutagenic, antiprogestational, antiprostatadenomic, antiprostatitic, antitumor, artemicide, bactericide, cancer preventive, candidicide, estrogenic, gonadotrophic, hypocholesterolemic, hypolipidemic, spermicide, viricide

425. SODIUM

426. STARCH: absorbent, antinesidioblastosic, emollient, poultice

427. STEARIC-ACID

428. ALPHA-P-DIMETHYL STYRENE

429. SUCROSE

430. DIETHYL-SULFIDE

431. ETHYL-ISOPROPYL-SULFIDE

432. METHYL-ALLYL-SULFIDE

433. 1-8-TERPINE HYDRATE

434. TERPINEN-4-OL: antiallergic, antiasthmatic, antiseptic, antitussive, bacteriostatic, fungicide, herbicide, insectifuge, spermicide

435. ALPHA-TERPINENE: insectifuge

436. GAMMA-TERPINENE: insectifuge

437. 4-TERPINEOL

438. ALPHA-TERPINEOL: termiticide

439. TERPINOLENE

440. TERPINOLENE EPOXIDE

441. ALPHA-TERPINYL ACETATE

442. THIAMIN: antialcoholic, antiberiberi, antocardiospasmic, anticolitic, antidecubitic, antideliriant, antiencephalopathic, antiheartburn, antiherpetic, antimigraine, antimyocarditic, antineaurasthenic, antineuritic, antipoliomyelitic, insectifuge

443. THREONINE: antiulcer

444. ALPHA-THUJENE

445. SESQUITHUJENE

446. BETA-THUJONE: insectifuge

447. TIN: antiacne, bactericide, taenicide

448. TOLUENE

449. TRICYCLENE

450. 2,2,4-TRIMETHYL-HEPTANE

451. TRYPTOPHAN: analgesic, antidepressant, antidyskinetic, antihypertensive, antimigraine, antiphenylketonutic, antipsychotic, antirheumatic, carcinogenic, hypnotic, insulinotonic, sedative, serotonigenic, tumor promoter

452. TYROSINE: antidepressant, antiencephalopathic, antiphenylketonuric, cancer preventive

453. UNDECAN-2-OL

454. AN-UNDECANONE

455. N-UNDECANONE

456. UNDECAN-2-ONE

457. VALERALDEHYDE

458. VALINE: antiencephalopathic

459. VANILLIC-ACID: antifatigue, anthelmintic, antioxidant, antisickling, ascaricide, bactericide, cancer preventive, choleretic, laxative

460. VANILLIN: allelochemic, cancer preventive, fungicide, insectifuge

461. VIT-B6

462. WATER

463. XANTHORRHIZOL

464. ALPHA-YLANGENE

465. BETA-YLANGENE

466. ZINGERONE: anti-inflammatory, cyclo-oxygenase inhibitor, hypotensive, 5-lipoxygenase inhibitor, paralytic, vasodilator

467. ZINGIBAIN: proteolytic

468. ZINC: antiacne, antiacrodermatitic, antianorexic, antiarthritic, anticoeliac, anticold, antidote (cadmium), antiencephalopathic, antifuruncular, antiherpetic, antiimpotence, antilepric, antiplaque, antistomatitic, antiulcer, antiulcer, antiviral, astringent, deodorant, immuno-suppressant, mucogenic, trichomonicide, vulnerary

469. ZINGIBERENE: antiulcer

470. ALPHA-ZINGIBERENE

471. BETA-ZINGIBERENE

472. ZINGIBERENOL

473. ZINGIBERINE

474. ZINGIBEROL

475. ZINGIBERONE

476. ZONARENE

477. ZT: hypocholesteremic

Notes of Reference
ⓖⓞⓞⓔ

The following references are listed
by chapter.

1. From the Start

1. a. Govindarajan, V. S. "Ginger — Chemistry, technology, and quality evaluation: Part 1." *Critical Reviews in Food Science and Nutrition* 17, no.1 (1982): 1-96 (p.1), citing Parry, J., *Spices*. Vols. 1 and 2, New York: Chemical Publishing Co., 1969.

   b. Ibid., 29.

2. McCaleb, R. S. "Rational Regulation of Herbal Products, Testimony before the Subcommittee on Government Operations." Herb Research Foundation, Washington, D.C., July 20, 1993.

3. Eisenberg, D. M., Kessler, R.C., Foster, C., Norlock, F. E., et al. "Unconventional medicine in the United States. Prevalence, costs, and patterns of use." *New England Journal of Medicine* 4 (28 Jan. 1993): 328; 246-52.

4. *Eating Well*, March-April 1993, 51.

2. From Cultivation to Confucius

1. Dahleen, M. "Ginger." *Horticulture* 57 (Nov. 1979): 24ff.

2. Rosengarten, *The Book of Spices*. Livingston Publishing Co., 1969, 257.

3. Purseglove, J. W., Brown, E.G., Green, C.L., Robbins, S.R.J. *Spices*. Vol. 2. London and New York: Longman Publishing, 1981, 449.

4. Thompson, E. H. et al. "Ginger rhizome: a new source of proteolytic enzyme." *Journal of Food Science* 38, no. 4 (1973): 652-55.

5. U.S. Department of Agriculture. *U.S. Spice Trade Circular Series*, April 1993.

6. Lawrence, B. "Major tropical spices — Ginger (*Zingiber officinale Rosc.*)." *Perfumer and Flavorist* 9 (Oct./Nov. 1984): 2-38 (p. 24).

7. Gladstar, R. *Healing Herbs for Women*. New York: Simon & Schuster, 1993, 243.

8. Rosengarten, *The Book of Spices*, 258.

9. See reference 1.

10. Govindarajan V.S. "Ginger—Chemistry, technology, and quality evaluation: Part 1." *Critical Reviews in Food Science and Nutrition* 17, no. 1 (1982): 1-96 (p.1).

11. Purseglove et al. *Spices*, 448.

12. Rosengarten, *The Book of Spices*, 259.

3. The Workings of a Miracle

1. Lawrence, B. "Major tropical spices — Ginger (*Zingiber officinale Rosc.*)." *Perfumer and Flavorist* 9 (Oct./Nov. 1984): 2-38 (p. 32).

2. Felter, H. W., and Lloyd, J. U. *King's American Dispensatory*. Portland, Ore.: Eclectic Medical, 1983, 2110.

3. Lawrence, "Major tropical spices," 35–36.

4. Govindarajan, V. S. "Ginger — chemistry, technology, and quality evaluation: Part 1." *Critical Reviews in Food Science and Nutrition* 17, no. 1 (1982): 1–96 (p. 50.)

5. Puri, H. S., and Pandey, G. "Glimpses into the crude drugs of Sikkim." *Bulletin Medical Ethnobotany Research* 1 (1980): 55–71.

6. Harborne, J. B., and Baxter, H., eds. *Phytochemical Dictionary: A Handbook of Bioactive Compounds from Plants*. Washington, D.C.: Taylor & Francis, 1993.

7. Govindarajan, "Ginger," 12.

8. Thompson, E. H., et al. "Ginger rhizome: A new source of proteolytic enzyme." *Journal of Food Science* 38, no. 4 (1973): 652-55.

9. Microsoft Bookshelf (1993). *Bartlett's Familiar Quotations* (licensed from Little, Brown & Co.) 1980: What I Have Learned [1966]. How Little I Know.

10. a. *Napralert Constituent Report*. Napralert Database, Chicago: College of Pharmacy, University of Illinois.

b. Duke, J. A. *Phytochemical Constituents of GRAS Herbs and Other Economic Plants* (Database). CRC Press, 1992.

c. See reference 3.

11. *Phytochemical Dictionary*, 481.

12. See reference 8.

13. a. Govindarajan, V. S. "Ginger — Chemistry, technology, and quality evaluation: Part 2." *Critical Reveiws in Food Science and Nutrition* 17, no. 3 (1982): 189-258 (p. 230), citing Huhtanen, C. "Inhibition of Clostridium botulinum by spice extracts and aliphatic alcohols." *Journal of Food Protection* 43, no. 3 (1980): 195.

b. Gugnani, H. C., and Ezenwanze, E. C. "Antibacterial activity of extracts of ginger and African oil bean seed." *Journal of Communicable Diseases* 17, no. 3 (Sept.): 233-36.

c. Mascolo, N., Jain, R., Jain, S. C., and Capasso, F. "Ethnopharmacologic investigation of ginger (*Zingiber officinale*)." *Journal of Ethnopharmacology* 27, nos. 1-2 (Nov. 1989): 129-40.

14. a. Adewunmi, C. O., Oguntimein, B. O., and Furu, P. "Molluscicidal and anti-schistosomal activities of *Zingiber officinale*." *Planta Medica* 56, no. 4 (Aug. 1990) 374-76.

b. Goto, C., Kasuya, S., Koga, K., Ohtomo, H., Kagei, N. "Lethal efficacy of extract from *Zingiber officinale* (traditional Chinese medicine) or [6]-shogaol and [6]-gingerol in Anisakis larvae in vitro." *Parasitology Research* 76, no. 8 (1990): 653-56.

c. Raj, R. "Screening of some indigenous plants for anthelmintic action against human ascaris lumbricoides." *Indian Journal Physiology and Pharmacology* 18, no. 2 (1974): 129-31.

d. Datta, A., and Sukal, N. "Antifilarial effects of *Zingiber officinale* on Dirofilaria immitis." *Journal of Helminthology* 61, (1987): 268-70.

e. Kiuchi, F. "Nematocidal activity of some anthelmintics, traditional medicines, and spices by new assay method using larvae of toxocara canis." *Shoyakugaku Zasshi* 43, no. 4 (1989): 279-87.

f. Ibid., citing Kucera, M. *Nigerian Journal of Pharmacy* 6 (1975): 77.

g. Ibid., citing Kucera, M., Kucerova, H. J. *Chromatography* 93 (1975): 421.

h. Ibid., citing Kucera, M., Theakston, R., Kucerova, H. *Nigerian Journal of Pharmacy* 6 (1975): 121.

i. Ibid., citing Adewunmi, C., Sofowora, E. A. *Planta Medica* 39 (1980): 57.

j. Ibid., citing Sukul, N., et al. "Nematicidal action of some edible crops." *Nematologica* 20: 187-91.

15. a. Kiuchi, F., and Shibuya, M., Sankawa, U. "Inhibitors of prostaglandin biosynthesis from ginger." *Chemical and Pharmaceutical Bulletin* (Tokyo) 30 (Feb. 1982): 754-57.

b. Mustafa, T., Srivastava, K. C. "Ginger and (*Zingiber officinale*) in migraine headache." *Journal of Ethnopharmacology* 29, no. 3 (July 1990): 267-73.

c. See reference 12c.

d. Srivastava, K. C., and Mustafa, T. "Ginger (*Zingiber Officinale*) in rheumatism and musculoskeletal disorders." *Medical Hypotheses* 39, no. 4 (Dec. 1992): 342-48.

e. Srivastava, K. C., and Mustafa, T. "Ginger (*Zingiber Officinale*) and rheumatic disorders." *Medical Hypotheses* 29, no. 1 (May 1989): 25-28.

f. Suekawa, M., Yuasa, K., Isono, M., Sone, H., et al. ["Pharmacological studies on ginger. IV. Effect of (6)-shogaol on the arachidonic cascade"] *Nippon Yakurigaku Zasshi (Folia Pharmacologica Japonica)* 88, no. 4 (Oct. 1986): 263-69.

g. Srivastava, K. C. "Effect of onion and ginger consumption on platelet thromboxane production in humans." *Prostaglandins, Leukotrienes and Essential Fatty Acids* 35, no. 3 (Mar. 1989): 183-85.

h. Srivastava, K. C. "Effects of aqueous extracts of onion, garlic and ginger on platelet aggregation and metabolism of arachidonic acid in the blood vascular system: In vitro study." *Prostaglandins, Leukotrienes and Medicine* 13 no. 2 (Feb. 1984): 227-35.

i. Srivastava, K. C. "Aqueous extracts of onion, garlic and ginger inhibit platelet aggregation and alter arachidonic acid metabolism." *Biomedica Biochimica Acta* 43, nos. 8-9: S335-46.

j. Srivastava, K. C. "Isolation and effects of some ginger components of platelet aggregation and eicosanoid biosynthesis." *Prostaglandins, Leukotrienes and Medicine* 25, nos. 2-3 (Dec. 1986): 187-98.

k. Flynn, D., et al. "Inhibition of human neutrophil 5 lipoxygenase activity by gingerdione, shogaol, capsaicin and related pungent compounds." *Prostaglandins, Leukotrienes and Medicine* 24 (1986): 195-98.

16. a. Rodeheaver, G., Marsh, D., Edgerton, M. T., abd Edlich, R.F. "Proteolytic enzymes as adjuncts to antimicrobial prophylaxis of contaminated wounds." *American Journal of Surgery* 129, no. 5 (May 1975): 537-44.

b. Baskanchiladze, G.S., Khurtsilava, L. A., Gelovani, I. A., Asatiani, M.V., and Rossinskii, V. I. "In combination with papain in experimental septicemia." *Antibiotiki* 29, no. 1 (Jan. 1984): 33-35.

c. Brisou, J., Babin, P., Babin, R. ["Potentialization of Antibiotics by lytic enzymes"]. Comptes; ["Chemotherapeutic effectiveness of antibiotics"] *Rendus des Seances de la Societe de Biologie et de Ses* 169, no. 3 (1975): 660-64.

d. Udod, V. M., Kolos, A. I., and Gritsuliak, Z. N. ["Treatment of patients with lung abscess by local administration of papain"] *Vestnik Khirurgii Imeni I. I. Grekova* 142, no. 3 (Mar. 1989): 24-27.

e. Emeruwa, A. C. "Antibacterial substance from Carica papaya fruit extract." *Journal of Natural Food Products* 45, no. 2 (Mar.-Apr. 1982): 123-27.

f. Neubauer, R. "A plant protease for potentiation of and possible replacement of antibiotics." *Experimental Medicine and Surgery* 19 (1961): 143-60.

17. a. See reference 16b.

18. Vogel, H. *The Nature Doctor.* New Canaan, Conn.: Keats Publishing, 1991, 446.

19. a. Taussig, S. J., and Batkin, S. "Bromelain, the enzyme complex of pineapple (ananas comosus) and its clinical application. An update." *Journal of Ethnopharmacology* 22, no. 2 (Feb.-Mar. 1988): 191-203.

b. Ito, C., Yamaguchi, K., Shibutani, Y., Suzuki, K., et al. ["Anti-inflammatory actions of proteases, bromelain, trypsin and their mixed preparation." *Nippon Yakurrigaku Zasshi [Folia Pharmacologica Japonica]* 75, no. 3 (Apr. 1979): 227-37.

c. Vellini, M., Desideri, D., Milanese, A., Omini, C., et al. "Possible involvement of eicosanoids in the pharmacological action of bromelain." *Arzneimittel-Forschung* 36, no. 1 (1986): 110-12.

20. a. Govindarajan, V. S. "Ginger — Chemistry, technology, and quality evaluation: Part 2." *Critical Reviews in Food Science and Nutrition* 17, no. 8 (1982): 189-258 (p. 230), *citing* Hirahara, F. "Antioxidative activity of various spices on oils and fats. Antioxidative activity towards oxidation on storage and heating." *Japanese Journal of Nutrition* 32, no. 1 (1974): 1; Food Sci Technol Abstr. 7, no. 3 (1975): T 126.

b. Saito, Y., Kimura, Y., and Sakamoto, T. "The antioxidant effects of petroleum ether soluble and insoluble fractions from spices." *Eiyo to Shokuryo* 29 (1976): 505-10.

c. Huang, J., et al. "Studies on the antioxidative activities of spices grown in Taiwan." *Chung-kuo Nung Yeh Hua Hsueh Hui Chih* 19 (1981): 3-4.

d. Lee, Chan Juan, et al. "Studies on the antioxidative activities of spices grown in Taiwan." *Chemical Abstracts* 97, no. 3 (1982).

e. Han, B., et al. "Chemical and Biochemical Studies on Antioxidant Components of Ginseng." *Advances in Chinese Medicinal Materials Research* (1985): 485-98.

f. Lee, Y. B., Kim, Y. S., and Ashmor, C. R. "Antioxidant property in ginger rhizome and its application to meat products." *Journal of Food Science* 51, no. 1 (1986): 20-23.

g. Ibid., citing Kihara, Y. and Inoue, T. "Antioxidant activity of spice powders in foods," citing *Chemical Abstracts* 59,

no. 19 (1961): 13, 276.

h. Ibid., citing Fujio et al. "Prevention of lipid oxidation in freeze-dried foods. Antioxidative effects of spices and vegetables." *Chemical Abstracts* 74 (1971): 2846.

i. Govindarajan, V. S. "Ginger — Chemistry, technology, and quality evaluation: Part 1." *Critical Reviews in Food Science and Nutrition* 17, no. 1 (1982): 1-96, citing Sethi, S. C., and Aggarwal, J. S. "Stabilization of edible fats by spices and condiments." *Journal of Scientific and Industrial Research* 1952; Sec. B11, 468.

j. Kikuzaki, H., and Nakatani, N. "Antioxidant effects of some ginger constituents." *Journal of Food Science* 58 (1993): 1407.

21. a. Vellini, M., Desideri, D., Milanese, A., Omini, C., et al. "Possible involvement of eicosanoids in the pharmacological action of bromelain." *Arzneimittel-forschung* 36, no. 1 (1986): 110-12.

b. Taussig and Batkin, "Bromelain, the enzyme complex of pineapple," 191-203.

c. Ito, C., Yamaguchi, K., Shibutani, Y., Suzuki, K., et al. ["Anti-inflammatory actions of proteases, bromelain, trypsin and their mixed preparation" (author's trans.)] *Nippon Yakurigaku Zasshi. [Folia Pharmacologica Japonica]* 75, no. 3 (20 Apr. 1979): 227-37.

d. Kiuchi, F., Iwakami, S., Shibuya, M., Hanaoka, F., and Sankawa, U. "Inhibition of prostaglandin and leukotriene biosynthesis by gingerols and diarylheptanoids." *Chemical and Pharmaceutical Bulletin* (Tokyo) 40, no. 2 (Feb.): 387-91.

22. a. Busse, W. W., and Gaddy, J. N. "The role of leukotriene antagonists and inhibitors in the treatment of airway disease." *American Review of Respiratory Disease* May 1991; 143 (5 Pt 2): S103-7.

b. Rask-Madsen, J., Bukhave, K., Laursen, L. S., and Lauritsen, K. "5-Lipoxygenase inhibitors for the treatment of inflammatory bowel disease." *Agents and Actions 1992*; Spec No: C37-46.

c. McMillan, R. M., and Walker, E. R. "Designing therapeutically effective 5-lipoxygenase inhibitors." *Trends in Pharmacological Sciences* 13, no. 8 (Aug. 1992): 323-30.

23. See reference 15d.

24. a. See reference 15d.

b. See reference 15e.

c. Hudson, N., Hawthorne, A. B., Cole, A. T., Jones, P. D., and Hawkey, C. J. "Mechanisms of gastric and duodenal damage and protection." *Hepato-Gastroenterology* 39 (Feb. 1992). Suppl. 1: 31-6.

d. Fiddler, G. I., and Lumley, P. "Preliminary clinical studies with thromboxane synthase inhibitors and thromboxane receptor blockers. A review." *Circulation* 81 (Jan. 1990) Suppl.: I69-78; discussion I79-80.

e. Hoet, B., et al. "Pharmacological manipulation of the thromboxane pathway in blood platelets." *Blood Circulation and Fibrinolysis* 1, no. 2 (June 1990): 225-33.

f. Gresele, P., et al. "Thromboxane synthase inhibitors, thromboxane receptor antagonists and dual blockers in thrombotic disorders." *Trends in Pharmacologial Sciences* 12, no. 4 (Apr. 1991): 158-63.

g. Backon, J. "Ginger: Inhibition of thromboxane synthetase and stimulation of prostacyclin. Relevance for medicine and psychiatry." *Medical Hypotheses* 20, no. 3 (July 1986): 271-78.

h. Wilson, D. E. "Role of prostaglandins in gastroduodenal mucosal protection." *Journal of Gastro-enterology* 13 (1991) Suppl. 1: S65-71.

i. Kimmey, M. B. "NSAIDs, ulcers, and prostaglandins." *Journal of Rheumatology* 19 (Nov. 1992) Suppl. 36: 68-73.

j. Dajani, E. Z., Wilson, D. E., and Agrawal, N. M. "Prostaglandins: An overview of the worldwide clinical experience." *Journal of the Association for Academic Minority Physicians* 2, no. 1 (1991): 23, 27-35.

k. Janusz, A. G., and Janusz, A. J. "Prostaglandins: Viable therapy in gastric ulceration." *South Dakota Journal of Medicine* 46, no. 2 (Feb. 1993): 45-47.

l. Cryer, B., and Feldman, M. "Effects of nonsteroidal anti-inflammatory drugs on endogenous gastrointestinal prostaglandins and therapeutic strategies for prevention and treatment of nonsteroidal anti-inflammatory drug-induced damage." *Archives of Internal Medicine* 152, no. 6 (June 1992): 1145-55.

m. Brzozowski, T. ["Gastroprotection in vivo and in vitro."] *Patolgia Polska* 43, no. 1 (1992): 1-9.

n. Camu, F., Van Lersberghe, C., and Lauwers, M. H. "Cardiovascular risks and benefits of perioperative nonsteroidal anti-inflammatory drug treatment." *Drugs* 44 (1992), Suppl. 5: 42-51.

25. See reference 24e.

26. See reference 24g.

27. Ylikorkala, O., and Viinikka, L. "The role of prostaglandins in obstetrical disorders." *Baillieres Clinical Obstetrics and Gynaecology* 6, no. 4 (Dec. 1992): 809-27.

28. Graham, N. M., Burrell, C. J., Douglas, R. M., Debelle, P., and Davies, L. "Adverse effects of aspirin and ibuprofen on immune function, viral shedding, and clinical status in rhinovirus-infected volunteers." *Journal of Infectious Diseases* 162, no. 6 (Dec. 1990): 1277-82.

29. McCredie, M., Ford, J. M., Taylor, J. S., and Stewart, J.H. "Analgesics and cancer of the renal pelvis in New South Wales." *Cancer* 49, no. 12 (15 June 1982): 2617-25.

30. a. See reference 24c.

    b. See reference 24h.

    c. See reference 24i.

    d. See reference 24j.

    e. See reference 24k.

    f. See reference 24l.

    g. See reference 24m.

    h. Bright-Asare, P., Habte, T., Yirgou, B., and Benjamin, J. "Prostaglandins, H2-receptor antagonists and peptic ulcer disease." *Drugs* 1988; 35 Suppl. 3:1-9.

31. See reference 15d.

32. See reference 24n.

33. a. Bailey, J. M., Low, C. E., and Pupillo, M. B. "Reye's syndrome and aspirin use: A possible immunological relationship." *Prostaglandins, Leukotrienes and Medicine* 8, no. 3 (Mar. 1982): 211-18.

    b. Kharazi, A. I., and Pishel', I. N. ["The role of arachidonic acid derivatives in the system of immunity and its changes in aging."] *Fiziologicheskii Zhurnal* 36, no. 1 (Jan.–Feb. 1990): 107-13.

    c. Thomsen, M. K., Ahnfelt-Ronne, I. ["Leukotrienes. A review of the significance for disease in man and the possibilities for therapeutic intervention."] *Ugeskrift for Laeger* 53, no. 3 (Jan. 14): 173-76.

    d. Droge, W., Wolf, M., Hacker-Shahin, B., et al. "Immunomodulatory action of eicosanoids and other small molecular weight products of macrophages." *Annali Dell Istituto Superiore Di Sanita* 27, no. 1 (1991): 67-69.

    e. Claesson, H. E., Odlander, B., and Jakobsson, P. J. "Leukotriene B4 in the immune system." *International Journal of Immunopharmacology* 14, no. 3 (1992): 441-49.

    f. Janniger, C. K., and Racis, S. P. "The arachidonic acid cascade: An immunologically based review." *Journal of Medicine* 18, no. 2 (1987): 69-80.

g. Rola-Pleszczynski, M. ["Regulation of the immune response using leukotrienes."] *Union Medicale du Canada* 118, no. 3 (May-June 1989): 111-13.

34. a. Schalin-Karrila, M., Mattila, L., Jansen, C. T., and Uotila, P. "Evening primrose oil in the treatment of atopic eczema: Effect on clinical status, plasma phospholipid fatty acids and circulating blood prostaglandins." *British Journal of Dermatology* 117, no. 1 (July 1987): 11-19.

b. el-Ela, S. H., Prasse, K. W., Carroll, R., Bunce, O. R., and Abou-el-Ela, S. H. "Effects of dietary primrose oil on mammary tumorigenesis induced by 7,12-dimethylbenz(a)anthracene." *Lipids* 22, no. 12 (Dec. 1987): 1041-44.

c. Belch, J. J., Shaw, B., O'Dowd, A., Saniabadi, A., et al. "Evening primrose oil (Efamol) in the treatment of Raynaud's phenomenon: A double blind study." *Thrombosis and Haemostasis* 54, no. 2 (Aug. 1985): 490-94.

d. Brzeski, M., Madhok, R., and Capell, H. A. "Evening primrose oil in patients with rheumatoid arthritis and side-effects of non-steroidal anti-inflammatory drugs." *British Journal of Rheumatology* 30, no. 5 (30 Oct. 1991): 370-72.

35. a. D'Almeida, A., Carter, J. P., Anatol, A., and Prost, C. "Effects of a combination of evening primrose oil (gamma linolenic acid) and fish oil (eicosapentaenoic + docahexaenoic acid) versus magnesium, and versus placebo in preventing pre-eclampsia." *Women and Health* 19, nos. 2-3 (1992): 117-31.

b. Bamford, J. T., Gibson, R.W., Renier, C. M. "Atopic eczema unresponsive to evening primrose oil (linoleic and gamma-linolenic acids)." *Journal of the American Academy of Dermatology* 13, no. 6 (1985): 959-65.

c. Khoo, S. K., Munro, C., and Battistutta, D. "Evening primrose oil and treatment of premenstrual syndrome [see comments]." *Medical Journal of Australia* 153, no. 4 (20 Aug. 1990): 189-92.

d. Greenfield, S. M., Green, A. T., Teare, J. P., Jenkins, A. P., et al. "A randomized controlled study of evening primrose oil and fish oil in ulcerative colitis." Alimentary Pharmacology and Therapeutics 7, no. 2 (Apr. 1993): 159-66.

e. Jantti, J., Seppala, E., Vapaatalo, H., and Isomaki, H. "Evening primrose oil and olive oil in treatment of rheumatoid arthritis." *Clinical Rheumatology* 8, no. 2 (June 1989): 238-44.

36. a. See reference 14a.

b. See reference 14b.

c. See reference 12c.

d. See reference 14d.

e. See reference 14e.

f. See reference 14f .

g. See reference 14h.

h. See reference 14i.

i. See reference 14j.

j. See reference 15k.

k. See reference 20d.

l. See reference 24g.

m. Umeda, M., et al. "Effects of certain herbal medicines on the biotransformation of arachidonic acid: A new pharmacological testing method using serum." *Journal of Ethnopharmacology* 23 (1988): 91-98.

37. a. See reference 13c.

b. See reference 15h.

c. See reference 15i.

38. See reference 15i.

39. See reference 15a.

40. a. See reference 15b.

b. See reference 15d.

c. See reference 15e.

d. Sertie, J., Basile, A., et al. "Preventive antiunlcer activity of the rhizome extract of *Zinger officinale.*" *Fitotherapia* 63 (1992): 155-59

e. Backon, J. "Ginger as an antiemetic: Possible side effects due to its thromboxane synthetase activity." [letter] *Anaesthesia* 46, no. 8 (Aug. 1991): 705-6.

f. Grontved, A., Brask, T., Kambskard, J., and Hentzer, E. "Ginger root against seasickness. A controlled trial on the open sea." *Acta Otolaryngologica* 105, nos. 1-2 (Jan.-Feb. 1988): 45-49.

g. Fischer-Rasmussen, W., Kjaer, S. K., Dahl, C., and Asping, U. "Ginger treatment of hyperemesis gravidarum." *European Journal of Obstetrics, Gynecology, and Reproductive Biology* 38, no. 1 (4 Jan. 1991): 19-24.

4. A Healer for 5,000 Years

1. Lad, V., and Frawley, D. *Yoga of Herbs.* Santa Fe: Lotus Press, 1986, 122.

2. Cost, B. *Ginger: East to West.* Reading, Mass.: Addison-Wesley, 1989, 67.

3. a. Lad and Frawley, *Yoga of Herbs*

b. Atal, C. K., Zutshi, U., and Rao, P.G. "Scientific evidence on the role of Ayurvedic herbals on bioavailability of drugs." *Journal of Ethnopharmacology* 4, no. 2 (Sept. 1981): 229-32

c. Sakai, Y., et al. "Effects of medicinal plant extracts from Chinese herbal medicines on the mutagenic activity of benzo(a)pyrene." *Mutation Research* 206 (1988): 327-34

4. Purseglove, J. W., Brown, E. G., Green, C. L., and Robbins, S.R.J. *Spices.* Vol. 2. London and New York: 1981, 447-532.

5. Cost, *Ginger, East to West.* 169.

6. Ody, P. *The Complete Medicinal Herbal.* London: Dorling Kindersley, 1993.

7. Swahn, J. O. *The Lore of Spices.* New York: Crescent Books (Outlet), 1991.

8. Cost, *Ginger,* 170.

9. Ibid., 146.

10. Ferguson, A. M. *All About Spices.* 1889, 131-45.

11. a.Lad and Frawley, *Yoga of Herbs*

b. Sakai, Y., et al. "Effects of medicinal plant extracts from Chinese herbal medicines on the mutagenic activity of benzo(a)pyrene." *Mutation Research* 206 (1988): 327-34.

12. Dahleen, M. "Ginger." *Horti-culture* 57, no. 1 (1979).

13. Felter, H. W., and Lloyd, J. U. *King's American Dispensatory.* Portland, Ore.: Eclectic Medical, 1983, 2111.

14. See reference 9.

15. Griggs, B. *Green Pharmacy,* Rochester, Vt.: Healing Arts Press, 127.

16. Beasley, J. D., and Swift, J. J. *The Kellogg Report. The Impact of Nutrition, Environment & Lifestyle on the Health of Americans.* Institute of Health Policy, Bard College, Annandale on Hudson, New York, 1989, 7G: 353.

17. Lee, Y. B., Kim, Y. S., and Ashmor, C. R. "Antioxidant property in ginger rhizome and its application to meat products." *Journal of Food Science* 51, no. 1 (1986): 20-23.

18. Holdsworth, D., and Wamoi, B. "Medicinal plants of the Admiralty Islands, Papua New Guinea. Part I." *International Journal of Crude Drug Research* 20, no. 4 (1982): 169-81.

19. Van Den Berg, M. A. "Ver-O-Peso: The ethnobotany of an Amazonian market." In *Advances in Economic Botany Ethnobotany in the Neotropics,* ed. G. T. Prance and J. A. Kallunki. New York Botanical Garden, 1984, 140-49.

20. Kiuchi, F., Shibuya, M., and Sankawa, U. "Inhibitors of prostaglandin biosynthesis from ginger." *Chemical and Pharmaceutical Bulletin* (Tokyo) 30, no. 2 (Feb. 1982): 754-57.

21. Lucas, R. *Secrets of the Chinese Herbalists.* New York: Parker Publishing Co., 1977.

22. Yamahara, J., Miki, K., Chisa-ka, T., and Sawada, T. "Cholagogic effect of ginger and its active constituents." *Journal of Ethnopharmacology* 13, no. 2 (May 1985): 217-25.

23. Roig, Y., and Mesa, J. T. *Plantas Medicinales, Aromaticas o Venenosas de Cuba.* Havana: Ministerio de Agricultura, 1945, 872 pp.

24. Liu, W. H. D. "Ginger root, a new antiemetic." *Anaesthesia* (U.K.) 45, no. 12 (1991): 1085ff.

25. Singh, Y. N. "Traditional medicine in Fiji: Some herbal folk cures used by Fiji Indians." *Journal of Ethnopharmacology* 15, no. 1 (1986): 57-88.

26. John, D. "One hundred useful raw drugs of the Kani tribes of Trivandrum Forest Division, Kerala, India." *International Journal of Crude Drug Research* 22, no. 1 (1984): 17-39.

27. Alam, M., et al. "Treatment of diabetes through herbal drugs in rural India." *Fitotherapia* 61,no. 3 (1990): 240-42.

28. Puri, H. S., and Pandey, G. "Glimpses into the crude drugs of Sikkim." *Bull Med Ethobot* 1 (1980): 55-71.

29. Rao, R. R., and Jamir, N. S. "Ethnobotanical studies in Nagaland. I. Medicinal plants." *Economic Botany* 36 (1982): 176-81.

30. Jain, S. K., and Tarafder, C. R. "Medicinal plant-lore of the Santals." *Economic Botany* 24 (1970): 241-78.

31. Comley, J. C. W. "New macrofilaricidal leads from plants?" *Tropical Medicine and Parasitology* 41, no. 1 (1990): 1-9.

32. Reddy, M. B., Rebby, K. R., and Reddy, M. N. "A survey of plant crude drugs of Anantapur District,

Andhra Pradesh, India." *International Journal of Crude Drug Research* 27, no. 3 (1989): 145-55.

33. Mustafa, T., and Srivastava, K. C. "Ginger (*Zingiber officinale*) in migraine headache." *Journal of Ethnopharmacology* 29, no. 3 (July 1990): 267-73.

34. Tanaka, S., Saito, M., and Tabata, M. "Bioassay of crude drugs for hair growth promoting activity in mice by a new simple method." *Planta Medica Supplement* 40 (1980): 84-90.

35. Hirschhorn, H. H. "Botanical remedies of the former Dutch East Indies (Indonesia). I. Eumycetes, pteridophyta, gymnospermae, angiosperme (monoctylendones only)." *Journal of Ethnopharmacology* 7, no. 2 (1983): 123-56.

36. Burkill, I. H. *Dictionary of the Economic Products of the Malay Peninsula.* Vol. 2. Kuala Lumpur, Malaysia: Ministry of Agriculture & Cooperatives, 1966.

37. Sussman, L. K. "Herbal medicine on Mauritius." *Journal of Ethnopharmacology* 2, (1980): 259-78.

38. Ishikura, N. "Flavonol glycosides in the flowers of hibiscus mutabilis f. versicolor." *Agricultural and Biological Chemistry* 46 (1982): 1705-6.

39. Adewunmi, C. O., Oguntimein, B. O., and Furu, P. "Molluscicidal and antischistosomal activities of *Zingiber officinale.*" *Planta Medica Supplement* 56, no. 4 (1990): 374-76.

40. Sofowora, A. "The present status of knowledge of the plants used in traditional medicine in Western Africa: A medical approach and a chemical evalua-

tion." *Journal of Ethnopharmacology* 2 (1980): 109-18.

41. Holdsworth, D. "Phytomedicine of the Madang Province, Papua New Guinea. Part I. Karkar Island." *International Journal of Crude Drug Research* 22, no. 3 (1984): 111-19.

42. Holdsworth, D., and Rali, T. "A survey of medicinal plants of the Southern Highlands, Papua New Guinea." *International Journal of Crude Drug Research* 27 no. 1 (1989): 1-8.

43. Holdsworth, D., Pilokos, B., and Lambes, P. "Traditional medicinal plants of New Ireland, Papua New Guinea." *International Journal of Crude Drug Research* 21, no. 4 (1983): 161-68.

44. a. See reference 42.

   b. See reference 41.

45. Ramirez, V. R., Mostacero, L. J., Garcia, A. E., Majia, C. F., et al. *Vegetales Empleados en Medicina Tradicional Norperuana.* Trujillo, Peru: Banco Agario del Peru & Nacl Univ Trujillo, June 1988, 54 pp.

46. Gonzalez, F., and Silva, M. "A survey of plants with antifertility properties described in the South American folk medicine." Abstr. Princess Congress I Bangkok Thailand, 10-13 December 1987, 20 pp.

47. Velazco, E. A. "Herbal and traditional practices related to maternal and child health-care." *Rural Reconstruction Review* (1980): 35-39.

48. Al-Yahya, M. A. "Phytochemical studies of the plants used in traditional medicine of Saudi Arabia." *Fitotherapia* 57, no. 3 (1986): 179-82.

49. a. See reference 20.

   b. Al-Yahya, M. A., Rafatullah, S., Mossa, J. S., Ageel, A. M., et al. "Gastro-protective activity of ginger, *Zingiber officinale rosc.*, in albino rats." *American Journal of Chinese Medicine* 17, nos. 1/2 (1989): 51-56.

50. a. See reference 48.

b. See reference 49b.

51. Woo, W. S., Lee, E. B., Shin, K. H., Kang, S. S., and Chi, H. J. "A review of research on plants for fertility regulation in Korea." *Korean Journal of Pharmacology* 12, no. 3 (1981): 153-70.

52. Hussein Ayoub, S. M., Baerheim-Suendsen, A. "Medicinal and aromatic plants in the Sudan: Usage and exploration." *Fitotherapia* 51 (1981): 243-46.

53. a. Haerdi, F. *Native Medicinal Plants of Ulanga District of Tanganyika (East Africa).* Dissertation, Verlag für Recht und Gesellschaft A G, Basel. Ph.D. Dissertation, Univ. Basel 1964.

b. Watt, J. M., and Breyer-Brandwijk, M. G. *The Medicinal and Poisonous Plants of Southern and Eastern Africa* (2d. ed.). London: E&S Livingstone Ltd., 1962.

54. Hantrakul, M., and Tejason, P. "Study of the acute toxicity and cardiovascular effects of ginger (*Zingiber officinale* roscoe)." *Thai Journal of Pharmaceutical Science* 1, no. 6 (1976): 517-30.

55. a. Panthong, A., and Tejasen, P. "Study of the effects and the mechanism of action of ginger (*Zingiber officinale roscoe*) on motility of the intact intestine in dogs." *Medical Bulletin* 14, no. 3 (1975): 221-31.

b. See reference 54.

c. Panthong, A., and Sivamogstham, P. "Pharmacological study of the action of ginger (*Zingiber officinale roscoe*) on the gastrointestinal tract." *Medical Bulletin* 13, no. 1 (1974): 41-53.

56. a. See reference 55a.

b. See reference 54.

57. Ketusinh, O., Wimolwattanpun, S., and Nilvises, N. "Smooth muscle actions of some Thai herbal carminatives." *Thai Journal of Pharmacology* 6, no. 1 (1984): 11-19.

58. Wasuwat, S. *A List of Thai Medicinal Plants, ASRCT, Bangkok.* ASRCT Research Report No. 1 on Res. Project. 17, 1967, 22 pp.

59. a. Loewsoponkul, P. *Effect of Thai Emmenagogue Drugs on Rat Uterine.* Master's Thesis, Univ. Bangkok, 1982, 96 pp.

b. See reference 57.

60. See reference 55c.

61. See reference 59a.

62. See reference 55a.

63. Grieve, M., Mrs. *A Modern Herbal.* Vol. I. New York: Dover Publications, 1971, 353-54.

64. *The Herbalist.* Hammond, Indiana: Hammond Book Co., 1931, 400 pp.

65. Kuts-Cheraux, A. W. *Naturàe Medicina & Naturopathic Dispensatory.* Yellow Springs, Ohio: Antioch Press, 1953, 279.

66. Ellingwood, F., and Lloyd, J. U. *American Materia Medica Therapeutics and Pharmacognosy.* Evanston, Ill. 279-80.

67. Morton J. F. "Current folk remedies of northern Venezuela." *Queensland Journal of Crude*

Drug Research 13 (1975): 97-121.

68. Petelot, A. *Les Plantes Medicinales du Cambodge, du Laos et du Vietnam.* Vols. 1-4. Archives des Recherches Agronomiques et Pastorales au Vietnam, no. 23, 1954.

69. Fleurentin, J., and Pelt, J. M. "Repertory of drugs and medicinal plants of Yemen." *Journal of Ethnopharmacology* 6, no. 1 (1982): 85-108.

70. Felter and Lloyd, *King's American Dispensatory.*

71. Kuts-Cheraux; *Naturie Medicina.*

72. Ellingwood and Lloyd, *American Materia.*

5. References for a Wonder Drug

1. Srivastava, K. C., and Mustafa, T. "Ginger (*Zingiber officinale*) and rheumatic disorders." *Medical Hypotheses* 29, no. 1 (May 1989): 25-28.

2. Srivastava, K. C., and Mustafa, T. "Ginger (*Zingiber officinale*) in rheumatism and musculoskeletal disorders." *Medical Hypotheses* 39, no. 4 (Dec. 1992): 342-48.

3. Beasley, J. D., and Swift, J. J. *The Kellogg Report. The Impact of Nutrition, Environment & Lifestyle on the Health of Americans.* Institute of Health Policy, Bard College, Annandale on Hudson, New York, 1989, 7G:353.

4. Murray, M., and Pizzorno, J. *Encyclopedia of Natural Medicine.* Rocklin, Calif.: Pima Publishing, 1991, 447.

5. Ibid., 492.

6. See reference 2.

7. a. Busse, W. W., and Gaddy, J. N. "The role of leukotriene antagonists and inhibitors in the treatment of airway disease." *American Review of Respiratory Disease* 143, 5 Pt. 2 (May 1991): S103-7.

b. Piacentini, G. L., and Kaliner, M. A. "The potential roles of leukotrienes in bronchial asthma." *American Review of Respiratory Disease* 143, 5 Pt. 2 (May 1991): S96-99.

c. Musser, J. H., and Kreft, A. F. "5-lipoxygenase: Properties, pharmacology, and the quinolinyl(bridged)aryl class of inhibitors." *Journal of Medicinal Chemistry* 35, no. 14 (10 July 1992): 2501-24.

8. a. Nattero, G., Allais, G., De Lorenzo, C., Benedetto, C., et al. "Relevance of prostaglandins in true menstrual migraine." *Headache* 29, no. 4 (Apr. 1989): 233-38.

b. Benedetto, C. "Eicosanoids in primary dysmenorrhea, endometriosis and menstrual migraine." *Gynecological Enocrinology* 3, no. 1 (1989): 71-94.

c. Vardi, Y., Rabey, I. M., Streifler, M., Schwartz, A., Lindner, H. R., and Zor, U. "Migraine attacks. Alleviation by an inhibitor of prostaglandin synthesis and action." *Neurology* 26, no. 5 (1976): 447-50.

d. Parantainen, J., Vapaatalo, H., and Hokkanen, E. "Relevance of prostaglandins in migraine." *Cephalalgia* 5 (May 1985) Suppl. 2: 93-97.

e. LaMancusa, R., Pulcinelli, F. M., Ferroni, P., Lenti, L., et al. "Blood leukotrienes in headache: Correlation with platelet activity." *Headache* 31, no. 6 (June 1991): 409-14.

f. Rabey, J. M., Vardi, Y., Van Dyck, D., and Streifler, M. "Ophthalmoplegic migraine: Amelioration by Flufenamic acid, a prostaglandin inhibitor." *Opthalmologica* 175, no. 3 (1977): 148-52.

9. *Townsend Letter for Doctors,* February/March 1993, citing *Family Practice News,* 15 October 1992.

9♦. a. Mascolo, N., Jain, R., Jain, S. C., and Capasso, F. "Ethnopharmacologic investigation of ginger (*Zingiber officinale*)." *Journal of Ethnopharmacology* 27, nos. 1-2 (Nov. 1989): 129-40.

b. Srivastava, K. C., and Mustafa, T. "Pharmacological effects of spices: Eicosanoid modulating activities and their significance in human health." *Bio Medical Reviews* (Bulgaria) 2 (1993): 15-29.

10. a. See reference 2.

b. See reference 1.

c. Mustafa, T., Srivastava, K. C., and Jensen, K. B. "Drug development report (9): Pharmacology of ginger, *Zingiber officinale.*" *J Drug Dev* 6, no. 1 (1993): 25-39.

11. Mustafa, T., and Srivastava, K. C. "Ginger (*Zingiber officinale*) in migraine headache." *Journal of Ethnopharmacology* 29, no. 3 (1990): 267-73.

12. Murray, M. T. *Natural Alternatives to Over-the-Counter and Prescription Drugs.* New York: Morrow, 1994, 383 pp., p. 69, citing Newman, N. M., and Ling, R.S.M. "Acetabular bone destruc-

tion related to non-steroidal anti-inflammatory drugs." *Lancet* 2 (1985): 11-13. Also citing Solomon, L. "Drug-induced arthropathy and necrosis of the femoral head." *Journal of Bone and Joint Surgery* 55 B (1973): 246-51. Also citing Ronningen, H., and Langeland, N. "Indomethacin treatment in osteoarthritis of the hip joint." *Acta Orthopeaedica Scandinavica* 50 (1979): 169-74.

13. See reference 11.

14. Public Citizen Health Research Group. 9, no. 4 (April 1993).

15. Joshua Backon, personal correspondence

16. See reference 12.

17. Beasley, J.D., and Swift, J.J. *The Kellogg Report. The Impact of Nutrition, Environment & Lifestyle on the Health of Americans.* Institute of Health Policy, Bard College, Annandale on Hudson, New York, 1989, 7D: 335.

18. Castleman, M. *An Aspirin A Day: What You Can Do to Prevent Heart Attack, Stroke, and Cancer.* New York: Hyperion, 1993, 4-5.

19. Dorso, C., et al. "Chinese food and platelets." *New England Journal of Medicine* 303, no. 13 (1980): 756-57.

20. Srivastava, K. C. "Effects of aqueous extracts of onion, garlic and ginger on platelet aggregation and metabolism of arachidonic acid in the blood vascular system: In vitro study." *Prostaglandins, Leukotrienes and Essential Fatty Acids* 13, no. 2 (Feb. 1984): 227-35.

21. The Aspirin Myocardial Infarction Study Research

Group. *"The aspirin myocardial infarction study: Final results."* *Circulation* 62 (6, Pt 2.) (Dec. 1980): V79-84

22. a. Srivastava, K. C. "Effect of onion and ginger consumption on platelet thromboxane production in humans." *Prostaglandins, Leukotrienes and Essential Fatty Acids* 35, no. 3 (Mar. 1989): 183-85.

b. See reference 20.

c. Srivastava, K. C. "Aqueous extracts of onion, garlic and ginger inhibit platelet aggregation and alter arachidonic acid metabolism." *Biomedica Biochimica Acta* 43, nos. 8-9 (1984): S335-46.

d. Srivastava, K. C. "Isolation and effects of some ginger components of platelet aggregation and eicosanoid biosynthesis." *Prostaglandins, Leukotrienes and Essential Fatty Acids* 25, nos. 2-3 (Dec. 1986): 187-98.

e. Kharazi, A. I., and Pishel', I. N. ["The role of arachidonic acid derivatives in the system of immunity and its changes in aging."] *Fiziologicheskii Zhurnal* 36, no. 1 (Jan.-Feb. 1990): 107-13.

f. Suekawa, M., et al. "Platelet aggregation inhibiting drug containing [6]-shogaol." *Chemical Abstracts* 109, no. 11 (1988).

g. Srivastava, K. C., and Mustafa, T. "Spices: Antiplatelet activity and prostanoid metabolism." *Prostaglandins, Leukotrienes and Essential Fatty Acids* 38 (1989): 255-66.

23. Verma, S.K., Singh, J., Khamesra, R., and Bordia, A. "Effect of ginger on platelet aggregation in man." *Indian Journal of Medical Research* 98 (1993): 240-42.

24. a. See reference 22a.

b. See reference 20.

c. See reference 22d.

25. a. Duke, J. "The joy of ginger." *American Health*, May 1988.

b. Ally, M. "The pharmacological action of *Zingiber officinale*." *Chemical Abstracts* 61 (1964): 6047.

c. Kobayashi, M., Ishida, Y., Shoji, N., and Ohizumi, Y. "Cardiotonic action of [8]-gingerol, an activator of the Ca++-pumping adenosine triphosphatase of sarcoplasmic reticulum, in guinea pig atrial muscle." *Journal of Pharmacology and Experimental Therapeutics* 246, no. 2 (Aug. 1988): 667-73.

d. Kobayashi, M., Shoji, N., and Ohizumi, Y. "Gingerol, a novel cardiotonic agent, activates the Ca2+-pumping ATPase in skeletal and cardiac sarcoplasmic reticulum." *Biochimica et Biophysica acta* 903, no. 1 (18 Sept. 1987): 96-102.

e. Shoji, N., Iwasa, A., Takemoto, T., Ishida, Y., and Ohizumi, Y. "Cardiotonic principles of Ginger (*Zingiber officinale roscoe*)." *Journal of Pharmaceutical Sciences* 71, no. 10 (1982): 1174-75.

26. a. Govindarajan, V. S. "Ginger—Chemistry, technology, and quality evaluation: Part 2." *Critical Reviews in Food Science and Nutrition* 17, no.

3 (1982): 189-258 (p. 230), citing Gujral, S., et al. "Effect of
Ginger (*Zingiber officinale
roscoe*) oleoresin on serum
and hepatic cholesterol levels
in cholesterol-fed rats."
*Nutrition Reports Interna-
tional* 17, no. 2 (1978): 183.

b. Tanabe, M., Chen, Y. D.,
Saito, K., and Kano, Y. "Cholesterol biosynthesis inhibitory component from *Zingiber
officinale roscoe.*" *Chemical
and Pharmaceutical Bulletin*
(Tokyo) 41, no. 4 (Apr. 1993):
710-13.

c. Giri, J., et al. *Medicinal &
Aromatic Plants Abstracts* 7,
no. 5 (1985).

27. Brody, J. "Vitamin E greatly
reduces risk of heart disease,
studies suggest best results found
in those taking large doses." *New
York Times*, 20 May 1993.

28. Citizens for Health Fax Hot-
line, 18, April 1994.

29. Sambaiah, K., and Srinivasan,
K. *Die Nahrung* 1 (1991): 47-51.

30. a. Yamahara, J., Miki, K.,
Chisaka, T., Sawada, T., et al.
"Cholagogic effect of ginger
and its active constituents."
*Journal of Ethnopharmacolo-
gy* 13, no. 2 (May 1985): 217-25.

b. See reference 9♦a.

c. Eldershaw, T.P.,
Colquhoun, E.Q., Dora, K.A.,
Peng, Z.C., and Clark, M.G.
"Pungent principles of ginger
(*Zingiber officinale*) are ther-
mogenic in the perfused rat
hindlimb." *International
Journal of Obesity* 16, no. 10
(Oct. 1992): 755-63.

d. Huang, Q., Matsuda, H.,
Sakai, K., Yamahara, J., and

Tamai, Y. ["The effect of ginger on serotonin-induced
hypothermia and diarrhea."]
*Yakugaku Zasshi (Journal
of the Pharmaceutical Society of Japan)* 110, no. 12
(Dec. 1990): 936-42.

e. Suekawa, M., Ishige, A.,
Yuasa, K., Sudo, K., et al.
"Pharmacological studies on
ginger. I. Pharmacological
actions of pungent constitutents, (6)-gingerol and (6)-
shogaol." *Journal of
Pharmacobio-Dynamics* 7,
no. 11 (1984): 836-48.

f. Onogi, T., Minami, M.,
Kuraishi, Y., and Satoh, M.
"Capsaicin-like effect of (6)-
shogoal on substance P-containing primary afferents of
rats: A possible mechanism of
its analgesic action." *Neuropharmacology* 31, no. 11
(1992): 1165-69.

g. Yamahara, J., Miki, K.,
Chisaka, T., Sawada, T., et al.
"Cholagogic effect of ginger
and its active constituents."
*Journal of Ethnopharmacol-
ogy* 13, no. 2 (1985): 217-25,
citing Stary, Z., "Über Erre-
gung der Warmenerven
durch Pharmaka." *Archiv für
Experimentelle Pathologie
und Pharmakologie* 105
(1925): 76-87.

h. Ibid., citing Jancsó-Gábor, A.,
and Szolcsányi, J. "Action of
rare earth metals complexes on
neurogenic as well as on
bradykinin-induced inflammation." *Journal of Pharmacy and
Pharmacology* 22 (1970): 366-71.

i. Ibid., citing Jancsó-Gábor,
A. "Anaesthesia-like condition and or potentiation of
hexobarbitol sleep produced

by pungent agents in normal and capsaicin-desensitized rats." *Acta Physiologica Academiae Scientiarum Hungaricae* 55 (1980): 57-62.

j. Ibid., citing Szolcsányi, J., and Jancsó-Gábor, A. "Capsaicin and other pungent agents as pharamacological tools in studies on thermoregulation." In *The Pharmacology of Thermoregulation and Drug Action*, ed. E. Schönbaum and P. Lomax. Basel: Karger, 1973, 395-409.

31. a. See reference 30c.

b. See reference 30d.

32. See reference 30c.

33. See reference 2.

34. a. Shiba, M., et al. "Antiulcer furanogermenone extraction from ginger." *Chemical Abstracts* 106, no. 6 (1987).

b. Yamahara, J., Hatakeyama, S., Taniguchi, K., Kawamura, M., and Yoshikawa, M. ["Stomachic principles in ginger. II. Pungent and anti-ulcer effects of low polar constituents isolated from ginger, the dried rhizoma of *Zingiber officinale Roscoe* cultivated in Taiwan. The absolute stereostructure of a new diarylheptanoid."] *Yakugaku Zasshi (Journal of the Pharmaceutical Society of Japan)* 112, no. 9 (Sept. 1992): 645-55.

c. Yamahara, J., Mochizuki, M., Rong, H. Q., Matsuda, H., and Fujimura, H. "The antiulcer effect in rats of ginger constituents." *Journal of Ethnopharmacology* 23, nos. 2-3 (July-Aug. 1988): 299-304.

d. Ibid., citing Ogiso, A., et al.

"Isolation and structure of an anti-peptic ulcer diterpene from a Thai medicinal plant." *Chemical and Pharmaceutical Bulletin* 26 (1978): 3117-23.

e. Al-Yahya, M. A., Rafatullah, S., Mossa, J. S., Ageel, A. M., et al. "Gastroprotective activity of ginger, *Zingiber officinale rosc.*, in albino rats." *American Journal of Chinese Medicine* 17, nos. 1-2: 51-56.

f. Ibid., citing Enchi et al. "Novel diterpenelactones with anti-peptic ulcer activity from Croton sublyratus." *Chemical and Pharmaceutical Bulletin* 28, no. 1 (1980) 227-34.

g. Ibid., citing Trease, E., and Evans, W. *Pharmacognosy* (11th ed.) London: Baillare Tindall, 1978, 632-37.

h. Wu, H., Ye, D., Bai, Y., and Zhao, Y. ["Effect of dry ginger and roasted ginger on experimental gastric ulcers in rats."] *Chung-Kuo Chung Yao Tsa Chih [Ching Journal of Chinese Material]* 15, no. 5 (May 1990): 278-80, 317-18.

i. Backon, J. "Ginger and carbon dioxide as thromboxane synthetase inhibitors: potential utility in treating peptic ulceration." *Gut* 28 (1987): 1323.

j. Sakai, K., et al. "Effect of extracts of Zingiberaceae herbs on gastric secretion in rabbits." *Chemical and Pharmaceutical Bulletin* 37, no. 1 (1989): 215-17.

k. Sertie, J., Basile, A., et al. "Preventive antiulcer activity of the rhizome extract of *Zingiber officinale*." *Fitotherapia* 63 (1992): 155-59.

l. Ibid., citing Gilbert, V.A.,

et al. *Hormone and Metabolic Research* 15 (1983): 320.

m. Yoshikawa, M., Hatakeyama, S., Taniguchi, K., Matuda, H., and Yamahara, J. "6-Gingesulfonic acid, a new anti-ulcer principle, and ginger- glycolipids A, B and C, three new monoacyldigalactosylglycerols from Zingiberis rhizoma originating in Taiwan." *Chemical and Pharmaceutical Bulletin* 40, no. 8 (1992): 2239-41.

n. Sertie, J., Basile, A., et al. "Preventive anti-ulcer activity of the rhizome extract of *Zingiber officinale.*" *Fito-therapia* 63 (1992): 155-59, citing Bennett T., *International Journal Tissue Reaction* 5 (1983): 237.

35. a. See reference 34a.

b. See reference 34b.

c. See reference 34c.

36. a. See reference 34l.

b. See reference 34m.

c. See reference 34n.

37. See reference 34k.

38. See reference 34e.

39. Bright-Asare, P., Habte, T., Yirgou, B., and Benjamin, J. "Prosta-glandins, H2-receptor antagonists and peptic ulcer disease." *Drugs* 35 (1988) Suppl. 3: 1-9.

40. Stec, L.F. "Peptic ulcer — The price of stress." *Bestways,* April 1980, 38-40.

41. "The 100 drugs by U.S. sales." *Medical Advertising News*, May 1993.

42. a. Chaturvedi, G.N., Mahadeo, P., Agrawal, A.K., and Gupta, J. P. "Some clinical and experimental studies on whole root of glycyrrhiza glabra linn. (yashtimadhu) in

peptic ulcer." *Indian Medical Gazette* 113 (1979): 200-205.

b. Rees, W. D., Rhodes, J., Wright, J. E., Stamford, L. F., and Bennett, A. "Effect of deglycyrrhizinated liquorice on gastric mucosal damage by aspirin." *Scandinavian Journal of Gastroenterology* 14, no. 5 (1979): 605-7.

c. Das, S. K., Das, V., Gulati, A. K., and Singh, V. P. "Deglycyrrhizinated liquorice in aphthous ulcers." *Journal of the Association of Physicians of India* 37, no. 10 (Oct. 1989): 647.

d. Morgan, A. G., McAdam, W. A., Pacsoo, C., and Darnborough, A. "Comparison between cimetidine and Caved-S in the treatment of gastric ulceration, and subsequent maintenance therapy." *Gut* 23, no. 6 (June 1982): 545-51.

e. Glick, L. "Deglycyrrhizinated liquorice for peptic ulcer" [letter]. *Lancet* 9, no. 2 (8302) (Oct. 1982): 817.

42♦. a. See reference 34j.

b. See reference 34k.

c. Koop, H., and Eissele, R. ["Reduction of gastric acid secretion: Pathophysiologic and clinically relevant sequelae."] Zeitschrift für Gastroenterologie 29, no. 11 (Nov. 1991): 613-17.

43. *U.S. News & World Report,* 21 February 1994.

44. Griggs, B. *Green Pharmacy*, Rochester, Vt.: Healing Arts Press 297, citing "Borderlines in Medical Science." Introductory lecture delivered at the Medical School of Harvard University, 6. Nov. 1861, in Medical Essays, 255 (p. 297).

45. a. See reference 30a.

b. Yamahara, J., Huang, Q. R., Li, Y.H., Xu, L., and Fujimura, H. "Gastrointestinal motility enhancing effect of ginger and its active constituents." *Chemical and Pharmaceutical Bulletin* 38, no. 2 (Feb. 1990): 430-31.

46. See reference 30a.

47. See reference 42c.

48. Thompson, E. H., et al. "Ginger Rhizome: A new source of proteolytic enzyme." *Journal of Food Science* 38 (1973): 652-55.

49. a. See reference 30a.

b. See reference 45b.

c. Yamahara et. al. "Gastroenterology Motility."

50. See reference 30a.

51. Nes, I. F., Skjekvale, R., et al. "The effect of natural spices and oleoresins on *Lactobacillus plantarum* and *Staphylococcus aureus*." *Microbial Associations and Interactions in Food*, 435-440.

52. Hikino, H., Kiso, Y., Kato, N., Hamada, Y., et al. "Antihepatotoxic actions of gingerols and diarylheptanoids." *Journal of Ethnopharmacology* 14, no. 1 (Sept. 1985): 31-39.

53. a. Yamahara, J., Rong, H.Q., Naitoh, Y., Kitani, T., and Fujimura, H. "Inhibition of cytotoxic drug-induced vomiting in suncus by a ginger constituent." *Journal of Ethnopharmacology* 27, no. 3 (Dec. 1989): 353-55.

b. Pace, J.C. "Oral ingestion of encapsulated ginger and reported self-care actions for the relief of chemotherapy-associated nausea and vomiting." *Dissertation Abstracts International (Sci)* 47, no. 8 (1987): 3297.

c. Liu, W.H. "Ginger root, a new antiemetic" [letter; comment]. *Anaesthesia* 45, no. 12 (Dec. 1990): 1085.

d. Backon, J. "Ginger as an antiemetic: Possible side effects due to its thromboxane synthetase activity [letter]." *Anaesthesia* 46, no. 8 (Aug. 1991): 705-6.

e. Grontved, A., Brask, T., Kambskard, J., and Hentzer, E. "Ginger root against seasickness. A controlled trial on the open sea." Acta Otolaryngologica 105, nos. 1-2 (Jan.-Feb. 1988): 45-49.

f. Mowrey, D. B., and Clayson, D. E. "Motion sickness, ginger, and psychophysics." *Lancet* 20, no. 1 (8273) (Mar. 1982): 655-57.

g. Grontved, A., and Hentzer, E. "Vertigo-reducing effect of ginger root. A controlled clinical study." *Journal of Oto-Rhino-Laryngology and Its Related Specialties* 48, no. 5 (1986): 282-86.

h. Backon, J. "Ginger in preventing nausea and vomiting of pregnancy; a caveat due to its thromboxane synthetase activity and effect on testosterone binding [letter]." *European Journal of Obstetrics, Gynecology, and Reproductive Biology* 42, no. 2 (1986): 163-64.

i. Bone, M. E., Wilkinson, D. J., Young, J. R., McNeil, J., and Charlton, S. "Ginger root—A new antiemetic. The effect of ginger root on postoperative nausea and vomiting after major gynaecological surgery." *Anaesthesia* 45, no. 8 (Aug. 1990): 669-71.

j. Phillips, S., Ruggier, R., and Hutchinson, S.E. "*Zingiber officinale* (ginger)—An antiemetic for day case surgery." *Anaesthesia* 48, no. 8 (1993): 715-17.

k. Fischer-Rasmussen, W., Kjaer, S.K., Dahl, C., and Asping, U. "Ginger treatment of hyperemesis gravidarum." *European Journal of Obstetrics, Gynecology, and Reproductive Biology* 38, no. 1 (Jan. 1991): 19-24.

54. a. *Physicians' Desk Reference.* 47th ed. Montvale, N. J.: Medical Economics, 1993, 1097.

b. Ibid., 2323.

55. See reference 45b.

56. a. Govindarajan, V. S. "Ginger—Chemistry, technology, and quality evaluation: Part 2." *Critical Reviews in Food Science and Nutrition* 17, no. 3 (1982): 189-258 (p. 230), citing Huhtanen, C. "Inhibition of Clostridium botulinum by spice extracts and aliphatic alcohols." *Journal of Food Protection* 43, no. 3 (1980): 195.

b. Gugnani, H. C., and Ezenwanze, E. C. "Antibacterial activity of extracts of ginger and African oil bean seed." *Journal of Communicable Diseases* 17, no. 3 (Sept. 1985): 233-36.

c. See reference 9✦a.

d. See reference 51.

57. a. Hudson, N., Hawthorne, A. B., Cole, A. T., Jones, P. D., and Hawkey, C. J. "Mechanisms of gastric and duodenal damage and protection." *Hepato-Gastroenterology* 39, Suppl. 1 (Feb. 1992): 31-36.

b. Brooks, W. S. "Short- and long-term management of peptic ulcer disease: Current role of H2-antagonists." *Hepato-Gastroenterology* 39, Suppl. 1 (Feb. 1992): 47-52.

58. See reference 51.

59. a. Isolauri, E., Juntunen, M., Rautanen, T., Sillanaukee, P., and Koivula, T. "A human Lactobacillus strain (Lactobacillus casei sp strain GG) promotes recovery from acute diarrhea in children." *Pediatrics* 88, no. 1 (July 1991): 90-97.

b. Motta, L., Blancato, G., Scornavacca, G., DeLuca, M., Vasquez, E., Gismondo, M. R., Lo Bue, A., and Chisari, G. ["Study on the activity of a therapeutic bacterial combination in intestinal motility disorders in the aged."] Clinica Terapeutica 138, no. 1 (15 July 1991): 27-35.

c. Sanders, M. E. "Summary of conclusions from a consensus panel of experts on health attributes of lactic cultures: Significance to fluid milk products containing cultures." *Journal of Dairy Science* 76, no. 7 (July 1993): 1819-28.

60. See reference 51.

61. See reference 53f.

62. a. Wood, C. D., Manno, J. E., et al. "Comparison of efficacy of ginger with various anti-motion sickness drugs." *Clinical Research Practices & Drug Regulatory Affairs* 6, no. 2 (1988): 129-36.

b. Stewart, J.J., Wood, M.J., Wood, C.D., and Mims, M.E. "Effects of ginger on motion sickness susceptibility and gastric function." *Pharmacology* 42, no. 2 (1991): 111-20.

63. See reference 53b.

64. See reference 53a.

65. See reference 53e.

66. See reference 53k.

67. See reference 53i.

68. See reference 53j.

69. *Physicians' Desk Reference.* 47th ed. 1952.

70. See reference 62.

71. a. See reference 53f.

b. See reference 53g.

72. a. See reference 34j.

b. See reference 62b.

73. See reference 53e.

73♦. See reference 45b.

74. a. See reference 30d.

b. See reference 45b.

c. Ibid.

d. Huang, Q. R., Iwamoto, M., Aoki, S.,Tanaka, N., et al. "Anti-5-hydroxytryptamine effect of galanolactone, diterpenoid isolated from ginger." *Chemical and Pharmaceutical Bulletin* (Tokyo) 39, no. 2 (Feb. 1991): 397-99.

75. a. Lumb, A. B. "Mechanism of antiemetic effect of ginger [letter]." *Anaesthesia* 48, no. 12 (Dec. 1993): 1118.

b. Tyers, M. B., and Freeman, A. J. "Mechanism of the anti-emetic activity of 5-HT3 receptor antagonists." *Oncology* 49, no. 4 (1992): 263-68.

76. Koltai, M., Mecs, I., and Kasa, M. "On the anti-inflammatory effect of sendai virus innoculation." *Archives of Virology* 67, no. 1 (1981): 91-95.

77. Karevina, T. G., Khokholia, V. P., Shevchuk, I. M. ["Effects of serotonin and stress on the state of the gastric mucosa in rats with the intact and transsected vagus nerve."] *Biulleten Eksperimentalnoi Biologii I Meditsiny* 108, no. 11 (Nov. 1989): 545-47.

78. Heistad, D. D., Harrison, D. G., and Armstrong, M. L. "Serotonin and experimental vascular disease." *International Journal of Cardiology* 14, no. 2 (Feb. 1987): 205-12.

79. Spannhake, E. W., Levin, J. L., Mellion, B. T., Gruetter, C. A., et al. "Reversal of 5HT-induced broncho-constriction by PGI2: Distribution of central and peripheral actions." *Journal of Applied Physiology: Respiratory, Environmental* 49, no. 3 (Sept. 1980): 521-27.

80. Lichtenthal, P. R., Wade, L. D., and Rossi, E. C. "The effect of ketanserin on blood pressure and platelets during cardiopulmonary bypass." *Anesthesia and Analgesia* 66, no. 11 (Nov. 1987): 1151-54.

81. a. See reference 78.

b. Schror, K., and Braun, M. "Platelets as a source of vasoactive mediators." *Stroke* 21, 12 Suppl. (Dec. 1990): IV 32-35.

82. See reference 45b.

83 a. Phillips, S., Hutchinson, S., and Ruggier, R. "*Zingiber officinale* does not affect gastric emptying rate: A randomised, placebo-controlled, crossover trial." *Anaesthesia* 48, no. 5 (1993): 393-95.

b. Suekawa, M., Ishige, A.,

Yuasa, K., Sudo, K., Aburada, M., and Hosoya, E. Pharmacological studies on ginger. I. Pharmacological actions of pungent constitutents, (6)-gingerol and (6)-shogaol. *Journal of Pharmacobio-Dynamics* 7, no. 11 (Nov. 1984): 836-48.

83.
a. Atal, C. K., Zutshi, U., and Rao, P. G. "Scientific evidence on the role of Ayurvedic herbals on bioavailability of drugs." *Journal of Ethnopharmacology* 4, no. 2 (Sept. 1981): 229-32.

b. Christopher, J. *School of Natural Healing*. Provo, Utah: Bi-World, 1976.

c. Motono, M. "Manufacture of topical cosmetics and pharmaceuticals containing ginger extracts as absorption accelerators." *Chemical Abstracts* 112 (1990): 2231-37.

84. See reference 75a.

85. Kawai, T., Kinoshita, K., Koyama, K., and Takahash K. "Antiemetic principles of Magnolia obovata bark and Singiber officinale shizome." *Planta Medica* 60, no. 1 (Feb. 1994): 17-20.

86. a. Atal, C. K., Zutsh, U., and Rao, P. G. "Scientific evidence on the role of Ayurvedic herbals on bioavailability of drugs." *Journal of Ethnopharmacology* 4, no. 2 (Sept. 1981): 229-32.

b. Christopher, J. *School of Natural Healing*. Provo Utah: Bi-World, 1976

c. Motono, M. "Manufacturer of topical cosmetics and pharmaceuticals containing ginger extracts as absorption accelerators." *Chemical Abstracts* 112 (1990): 2231-37.

87. See reference 86a.

88. Srivastava, K. C., and Mustafa, T. "Ginger (*Zingiber officinale*) in rheumatism and musculoskeletal disorders." *Medical Hypotheses* 39, no. 4 (Dec. 1992): 342-48, citing Dorso, C., et al., "Chinese food and platelets." *New England Journal of Medicine* 303 (1980): 756-57.

89. See reference 86b.

90. See reference 86c.

91. a. Adewunmi, C. O., Oguntimein, B. O., and Furu, P. "Molluscicidal and antischistosomal activities of *Zingiber officinale*." *Planta Medica* 56, no. 4 (Aug. 1990): 374-76.

b. Goto, C., Kasuya, S., Koga, K., Ohtomo, H., and Kagei, N. "Lethal efficacy of extract from *Zingiber officinale* (traditional Chinese medicine) or [6]-shogaol and [6]-gingerol in Anisakis larvae in vitro." *Parasitology Research* 76, no. 8 (1990): 653-56.

c. Raj, R. "Screening of some indigenous plants for anthelmintic action against human ascaris lumbricoides." *Indian Journal Physiology and Pharmacology* 18, no. 2 (1974): 129-31.

d. Datta, A., and Sukal, N. "Antifilarial effects of *Zingiber officinale* on Dirofilaria immitis." *Journal of Helminthology* 61 (1987): 268-70.

e. Kiuchi, F. "Nematocidal activity of some anthelmintics, traditional medicines, and spices by new assay method using larvae of toxocara canis." *Shoyakugaku Zasshi* 43, no. 4 (1989): 279-87.

f. Ibid., citing Kucera, M.

Nigerian Journal of Pharmacy 6 (1975): 77.

g. Ibid., citing Kucera, M., and Kucerova, H. J. *Chromatography* 93 (1975): 421.

h. Ibid., citing Kucera, M., Theakston, R., and Kucerova, H. *Nigerian Journal of Pharmacy* 6 (1975): 121.

i. Ibid., citing Adewunmi, C., and Sofowora, E. A. *Planta Medica* 39 (1980): 57.

j. Ibid., citing Sukul, N., et al. "Nematicidal action of some edible crops." *Nematologica* 20: 187-91.

92. Brody, Jane, *New York Times*, 1 April 1993.

93. Dalton, H. P., and Nottebart, H. C., Jr. *Interpretative Medical Microbiology* (1986): 501.

94. a. Feroz, H., et al. "Review of scientific studies of anthelmintics from plants." *Journal of Sc Res on Pl & Med* 3 (1982): 1, 6-12.

    b. Tietze, P. E., and Tietze, P. H. "The roundworm, Ascaris lumbricoides." *Primary Care; Clinics in Office Practice* 18, no. 1 (Mar. 1991): 25-41.

95. Markell, E. K. et al., *Medical Parasitology.* 6th ed. Philadelphia: Saunders, 1986, 165.

96. Ibid., 166.

97. a. See reference 94b.

    b. Raj, R. "Screening of some indigenous plants for anthelmintic action against human ascaris lumbricoides." *Indian Journal Physiology and Pharmacology* 18, no. 2 (1974): 129-31.

98. Markell, et al.Voge, M., *Medical Parasitology*, 243.

99. See reference 91d.

100. Markell, et al. *Medical Parasitology.* 167.

101. Capron, A. R. "Immunity to schistosomes." *Current Opinion in Immunology* 4, no. 4 (Aug. 1992): 419-24.

102. Markell et al. *Medical Parasitology*, 167.

103. See reference 91a.

104. See reference 91h.

105. See reference 2.

106. a. See reference 56a.

     b. See reference 56b.

     c. See reference 9♦a.

107. Dean, M., Dhaliwal, A., and Jones, W. "Effects of *Zingiberacae* rhizome extract on the infectivity of cyanophage LPP-1." *Transactions of the Illinois State Academy of Science* 80: April 10-12, 1987.

108. a. Endo, K., et al. "Structures of antifungal diarylheptenones, gingerenones A, B, C and isogingerenone B, isolated from the rhizomes of *Zingiber officinale.*" *Phytochemistry* 29, no. 3 (1990): 797-99.

     b. Govindarajan, V. S. "Ginger—Chemistry, technology, and quality evaluation: Part 2." *Critical Reviews in Food Science and Nutrition* 17, no. 3 (1982): 189-258 (p. 230), citing Hitokoto, H., et al. "Inhibitory effects of spices on growth and toxin production of toxigenic fungi." *Applied and Environmental Microbiology* 39, no. 4 (1980): 818.

     c. Guérin, J. C., and Réveillère, H. P. "Activité antifongique d'extraits végétaux à usage thérApeutique 1."

Etude de 41 extraits sur 9 souches fongiques." *Ann Pharmaceutiques Françaises* 42, no. 6 (1984): 553-59.

109. a. See reference 25a.

b. Yamazaki, M., and Nishimura, T. "Induction of neutrophil accumulation by vegetable juice." *Bioscience Biotechnology Biochemistry* 1 (1992): 150-51.

110. "Antihistaminic substance from ginger." *Toyoda Isao* (Japan) 69 (21 Apr. 1969): 08, 561 (*Chemical Abstracts*).

111. See reference 30e.

112. *Microsoft Bookshelf, The Concise Columbia Dictionary of Quotations*, New York: Columbia University Press, 1990.

113. Ames, B. "Dietary carcinogens and anticarcinogens." *Science* 23 (Sept. 1983): 1256-64.

114. Morita, S., et al. "Studies on natural desmutagens: Screening for vegetable and fruit factors active in activation of mutagenic pyrolysis products from amino acids." *Agricultural and Biological Chemistry* 42, no. 6 (1978): 1235-38.

115. Yamaguchi, T. "Desmutagenic activity of peroxidase on autoxidized linolenic acid." *Agricultural and Biological Chemistry* 44, no. 4 (1980): 959-61.

115♦ a. Sakai, Y., et al. "Effects of medicinal plant extracts from Chinese herbal medicines on the mutagenic activity of benzo(a)pyrene." *Mutation Research* 206 (1988): 327-34.

b. See reference 114.

c. Nakamura, H., and Yamamoto, T. "Mutagen and anti-mutagen in ginger, *Zingiber officinale*." *Mutation*

Research 103, no. 2 (Feb. 1982): 119-26.

d. Sakai, Y. et al. "Effects of medicinal plant extracts from Chinese herbal medicines on the mutagenic activity of benzo(a)pyrene." *Mutation Research* 206 (1988): 327-34.

e. Kada, T., Morita, M., and Inoue, T. "Antimutagenic action of vegetable factor(s) on the mutagenic principle of tryptophan pyrolysate" *Mutation Research* 53 (1978): 351-53.

f. See reference 115.

g. Nagabhushan, M., Amonkar, A. J., and Bhide, S. V. "Mutagenicity of gingerol and shogaol and antimutagenicity of zingerone in Salmonella/-microsome assay." *Cancer Letters* 36, no. 2 (Aug. 1987): 221-33.

115□. a. Unnikrihnan, M. "Tumour reducing and anticarcinogenic activity of selected spices." *Cancer Letters* 51 (1990): 85-89.

b. Ibid., citing Unnikrihnan, M., and Kuttan, R. "Cytotoxicity of extracts of spices to cultured cells." *Nutrition and Cancer* 11, no. 4 (1988): 251.

c. Ibid., citing Goodpasture, C., and Arrighi, F. "Effects of food seasoning on the cycle and chromosomemorphology of mamalian cells in vitro with special reference to turmeric." *Food and Cosmetic Toxicology* 14 (1976): 2.

116. See reference 115□a.

117. Ohta, S., et al. "Studies on chemical protectors against radiation. XXV. Radioprotective activi-

ties of various crude drugs." *Yaku-gaku Zasshi* 107, no. 1 (1987): 70-75.

118. Wu, H., Cai, B. C., Shi, X. L., and Ye, D. J. ["The effect of stimulation and toxicity of rhizoma Pinelliae processed by ginger juice on animals."] *Chung-Kuo Chung Yao Tsa Chih [China Journal of Chinese Materia]* 18, no. 7 (July 1993): 408-10, 446-47.

119. Castleman, M. *An Aspirin a Day: What You Can Do to Prevent Heart Attack, Stroke, and Cancer.* New York: Hyperion, 1993, 79.

120. Mascolo, N., Jain, R., Jain, S. C., and Capasso, F. "Ethnopharmacologic investigation of ginger (*Zingiber officinale*)." *Journal of Ethnopharmacology* 27, nos. 1-2 (Nov. 1989): 129-40.

121. a. Duke, J. "The joy of ginger." *American Health,* May 1988.

b. Yamazaki, M., and Nishimura, T. "Induction of neutrophil accumulation by vegetable juice." *Bioscience Biotechnology Biochemistry* 1 (1992): 150-51.

122. See reference 121b.

123. a. Agarwal, K. C., and Parks, R. E. "Forskolin: A potential antimetastatic agent." *International Journal of Cancer* 32 (1983): 801-4.

b. Tzanakakis, G. N., Agarwal, K. C., and Vezeridis, M. P. "Prevention of human pancreatic cancer cell-induced hepatic metastasis in nude mice by dipyridamole and its analog RA-233." *Cancer* 71, no. 8 (Apr. 1993): 2466-71.

c. Tzanakakis, G. N., Agarwal, K. C., and Vezeridis, M. P. "Inhibition of hepatic metastasis from a human pancreat-ic adenocarcinoma (RWP-2) in the nude mouse by prostacyclin, forskolin, and ketoconazole." *Cancer* 65, no. 3 (Feb. 1990): 446-51.

d. Tzanakakis, G. N., Agarwal, K. C., Veronikis, D. K., and Vezeridis, M. P. "Effects of antiplatelet agents alone or in combinations on platelet aggregation and on liver metastases from a human pancreatic adenocarcinoma in the nude mouse." *Journal of Surgical Oncology* 48 (1991): 45-50.

124. a. See reference 115♦c.

b. See reference 115♦g.

125. See reference 9♦.

126. a. Govindarajan, V. S. "Ginger—Chemistry, technology, and quality evaluation: Part 2." *Critical Reviews in Food Science and Nutrition* 17, no. 3 (1982): 189-258 (p. 230), citing Gujral, S., et al. "Effect of ginger (*Zingiber officinale Roscoe*) oleoresin on serum and hepatic cholesterol levels in cholesterol-fed rats." *Nutr Rep Int* 17, no. 2 (1978): 183.

b. Tanabe, M., Chen, Y. D., Saito, K., and Kano, Y. "Cholesterol biosynthesis inhibitory component from *Zingiber officinale Roscoe*." *Chemical and Pharmaceutical Bulletin* (Tokyo) 41, no. 4 (Apr. 1993): 710-13.

c. Giri, J., et al. *Medicinal and Aromatic Plants Abstracts* 7 (1985): 5.

127. a. Ally, M. "The pharmacological action of *Zingiber officinale*." *Chemical Abstracts* 61 (1964): 6047.

b. Kobayashi, M., Ishida, Y., Shoji, N., and Ohizumi, Y. "Cardiotonic action of [8]-gingerol, an activator of the Ca++-pumping adenosine triphosphatase of sarcoplasmic reticulum, in guinea pig atrial muscle." *Journal of Pharmacology and Experimental Therapeutics* 246, no. 2 (Aug. 1988): 667-73.

c. Kobayashi, M., Shoji, N., Ohizumi, Y. "Gingerol, a novel cardiotonic agent, activates the Ca2+-pumping ATPase in skeletal and cardiac sarcoplasmic reticulum." *Biochimica et Biophysica Acta* 903, no. 1 (Sept. 1993): 96-102.

d. Shoji, N., Iwasa, A., Takemoto, T., Ishida, Y., and Ohizumi, Y. "Cardiotonic principles of ginger (*Zingiber officinale Roscoe*)." *Journal of Pharmaceutical Sciences* 71, no. 10 (Oct 1982): 1174-75.

128. a. See reference 30e.

b. See reference 127a.

c. Yamahara, J., Miki, K., Chisaka, T., Sawada, T., et al. "Cholagogic effect of ginger and its active constituents." *Journal of Ethnopharmacology* 13, no. 2 (May 1985): 217-25, citing Kasahara, Y., et al. "Pharmacological actions of Pinellia Tubers and *Zingiber* rhizomes." *Shoyakugaku Zasshi* 37 (1985): 73-83.

129. a. See reference 25a.

b. Yamazaki, M., and Nishimura, T. "Induction of neutrophil accumulation by vegetable juice." *Bioscience Biotechnology Biochemistry* 1 (1992): 150-51.

130. a. Backon, J. "Possible utility of a thromboxane synthetase inhibitor in preventing penile vascular changes and impotence during aging." *Archives of Andrology* 20 (1988): 101-2.

b. Backon, J. "Mechanism of analgesic effect of clonidine in the treatment of dysmenorrhea." *Medical Hypotheses* 36, no. 3 (Nov. 1991): 223-24.

c. Xiong, H. X. ["Changes in multihormones in treating male sterility with acupuncture and indirect moxibustion using ginger slices on the skin."] *Chung Hsi I Chieh Ho Tsa Chih* 6, no. 12 (Dec. 1986): 726-27, 708.

d. Cai, R., Zhou, A., and Gao, H. ["Study on correction of abnormal fetal position by applying ginger paste at zhihying acupoint A. Report of 133 cases."] *Chen Tzu Yen Chiu [Acupuncture Research]* 15, no. 2 (1990): 89-91.

131. Qureshi, S., Shah, A. H., Tariq, M., and Ageel, A. M. "Studies on herbal aphrodisiacs used in Arab system of medicine." *American Journal of Chinese Medicine* 17, nos. 1- 2 (1989): 57-63.

132. See reference 130d.

133. See reference 130a.

134. See reference 130b.

6. Charting Ginger's Accomplishments

1. Backon, J. "Ginger: Inhibition of thromboxane synthetase and stimulation of prostacyclin: Relevance for medicine and psychiatry." *Medical Hypotheses* 20, no. 3 (July 1986): 271-78.

2. Srivastava, K. C. "Effects of aqueous extracts of onion, garlic and ginger on platelet aggregation and metabolism of arachidon-

ic acid in the blood vascular system: In vitro study." *Prostaglandins Leukotrienes and Medicine* 13, no. 2 (1984): 227-35.

3. Srivastava, K. C. "Effect of onion and ginger consumption on platelet thromboxane production in humans." *Prostaglandins, Leukotrienes and Essential Fatty Acids* 35, no. 3 (Mar. 1989): 183-85.

4. Mascolo, N., Jain, R., Jain, S. C., and Capasso, F. "Ethnopharmacologic investigation of ginger (*Zingiber officinale*)." *Journal of Ethnopharmacology* 27, nos. 1-2 (Nov. 1989): 129-40.

5. Srivastava, K. C., and Mustafa, T. "Ginger (*Zingiber officinale*) in rheumatism and musculoskeletal disorders." *Medical Hypotheses* 39, no. 4 (Dec. 1992): 342-48.

6. Lee, Y. B., Kim, Y. S., and Ashmor, C. R. "Antioxidant property in Ginger Rhizome and its application to meat products." *Journal of Food Science* 51, no. 1 (1986): 20-23.

7. Saito, Y., Kimura, Y., and Sakamoto, T. "The antioxidant effects of petroleum ether soluble and insoluble fractions from spices." *Eiyo to Shokuryo* 29 (1976): 505-10.

8. Yamahara, J., Huang, Q. R., Li, Y. H., Xu, L., and Fujimura, H. "Gastrointestinal motility enhancing effect of ginger and its active constituents." *Chemical and Pharmaceutical Bulletin* 38, no. 2 (Feb. 1990): 430-31.

9. Sakai, K., et al. "Effect of extracts of *Zingiberaceae* herbs on gastric secretion in rabbits." *Chemical and Pharmaceutical Bulletin* 37, no. 1 (1989): 215-17.

10. Sertie, J., Basile, A., et al. "Preventive anti-ulcer activity of the rhizome extract of *Zingiber officinale*." *Fitoterapia*

63 (1992): 155-59.

11. Al-Yahya, M. A., Rafatullah, S., Mossa, J. S., Ageel, A. M., et al. "Gastroprotective activity of ginger, *Zingiber officinale rosc.*, in albino rats." *American Journal of Chinese Medicine* 17, nos. 1-2 (1989): 51-56.

12. See reference 10.

13. "The 100 drugs by U.S. sales." *Medical Advertising News*, May 1993.

14. Qureshi, S., Shah, A. H., Tariq, M., and Ageel, A. M. "Studies on herbal aphrodisiacs used in Arab system of medicine." *American Journal of Chinese Medicine* 17, nos. 1-2 (1989): 57-63.

7. Give Me My Ginger

1. a. Govindarajan, V. S. "Ginger — Chemistry, technology, and quality evaluation: Part 1." *Critical Reviews in Food Science and Nutrition* 17, no. 1 (1982): 1-96 (p. 4).

b. Ibid., 21, citing Scott, P., and Kennedy, R. "Analysis of spices and herbs for aflatoxins." *Canadian Institute of Food Science and Technology Journal* 8, no. 2 (1975): 124.

c. Ibid., 23.

d. Ibid., 26.

e. Ibid., 28.

2. a. Yamahara et al. "Active components of ginger exhibiting antiserotonergic action." *Phytotherapy Research* 3, no. 2 (1989): 70-71.

b. Huang, Q., Matsuda, H., Sakai, K., Yamahara, J., and Tamai, Y. ["The effect of ginger on serotonin-induced hypothermia and diarrhea."]

Yakugaku Zasshi [Journal of the Pharmaceutical Society of Japan] 110, no. 12 (Dec. 1990): 936-42.

3. Flynn, D., et al. "Inhibition of human neutrophil 5 lipoxygenase activity by gingerdione, shogaol, capsaicin and related pungent compounds." *Prostaglandins, Leukotrienes and Medicine* 24 (1986): 195-98.

4. Kiuchi, F., Shibuya, M., and Sankawa, U. "Inhibitors of prostaglandin biosynthesis from ginger." *Chemical and Pharmaceutical Bulletin* (Tokyo) 30, no. 2 (Feb. 1982): 754-57.

5. Suekawa, M., Ishige, A., Yuasa, K., Sudo, K., et al. "Pharmacological studies on ginger. I. Pharmacological actions of pungent constitutents, (6)-gingerol and (6)-shogaol." *Journal of Pharmacobio-dynamics* 7, no. 11 (Nov. 1984): 836-48.

6. a. Adewunmi, C. O., Oguntimein, B. O., and Furu, P. "Molluscicidal and antischistosomal activities of *Zingiber officinale*." *Planta Medica* 56, no. 4 (Aug. 1990): 374-76.

b. Goto, C., Kasuya, S., Koga, K., Ohtomo, H., and Kagei, N. "Lethal efficacy of extract from *Zingiber officinale* (traditional Chinese medicine) or [6]-shogaol and [6]-gingerol in Anisakis larvae in vitro." *Parasitology Research* 76, no. 8 (1990): 653-56.

7. See reference 2b.

8. Yamahara, J., Rong, H. Q., Naitoh, Y., Kitani, T., and Fujimura, H. "Inhibition of cytotoxic drug-induced vomiting in suncus by a ginger constituent." *Journal of Ethnopharmacology*

27, no. 3 (1989): 353-55.

9. Kawai, T., Kinoshita, K., Koyama, K., and Takahashi, K. "Antiemetic principles of Magnolia obovata bark and *Zingiber officinale* rhizome." *Planta Medica* 60, no. 1 (Feb. 1994): 17-20.

10. *Phytochemistry Dictionary: A Handbook of Bioactive Compounds from Plants.* Harborne, J. B., and Baxter, H., eds.Washington, D.C.: Taylor & Francis, 1993, 481.

11. Hikino, H., Kiso, Y., Kato, N., Hamada, Y., Shioiri, T., Aiyama, R., Itokawa, H., Kiuchi, F., and Sankawa, U. "Antihepatotoxic actions of gingerols and diarylheptanoids." *Journal of Ethnopharmacology* 14, no. 1 (Sept. 1985): 31-39.

12. Lad, V., and Frawley, D. *Yoga of Herbs.* Santa Fe, N. M.: Lotus Press, 1986, 122.

13. Yamahara, J., Mochizuki, M., Rong, H. Q., Matsuda, H., and Fujimura, H. "The antiulcer effect in rats of ginger constituents." *Journal of Ethnopharmacology* 23, no. 2 (July–Aug. 1988): 299-304.

14. Yamahara, J., Hatakeyama, S., Taniguchi, K., Kawamura, M., and Yoshikawa, M. ["Stomachic principles in ginger. II. Pungent and anti-ulcer effects of low polar constituents isolated from ginger, the dried rhizoma of *Zingiber officinale* Roscoe cultivated in Taiwan. The absolute stereostructure of a new diarylheptanoid."] *Yakugaku Zasshi [Journal of the Pharmaceutical Society of Japan]* 112, no. 9 (Sept. 1992): 645-55.

15. Kobayashi, M., Shoji, N., and Ohizumi, Y. "Gingerol, a novel cardiotonic agent, activates the $Ca2+$-pumping ATPase in skeletal and cardiac sarcoplasmic reticulum."

Biochimica et Biophysica Acta 903, no. 1 (Sept. 1987): 96-102.

16. Yamahara, J., Huang, Q. R., Li, Y. H., Xu, L., and Fujimura, H. "Gastrointestinal motility enhancing effect of ginger and its active constituents." *Chemical and Pharmaceutical Bulletin* 38, no. 2 (Feb. 1990): 430-31.

17. Eldershaw, T. P., Colquhoun, E. Q., Dora, K. A., Peng, Z. C., and Clark, M. G. "Pungent principles of ginger (*Zingiber officinale*) are thermogenic in the perfused rat hindlimb." *International Journal of Obesity* 16, no. 10 (Oct. 1992): 755-63.

18. See note 11.

19. See reference 6a.

20. a. Suekawa, M., Ishige, A., Yuasa, K., Sudo, K., et al. "Pharmacological studies on ginger. I. Pharmacological actions of pungent constitutents, (6)-gingerol and (6)-shogaol." *Journal of Pharmacobio-dynamics* 7, no. 11 (Nov. 1984): 836-48.

b. Onogi, T., Minami, M., Kuraishi, Y., and Satoh, M. "Capsaicin-like effect of (6)-shogoal on substance P-containing primary afferents of rats: A possible mechanism of its analgesic action." *Neuropharmacology* 31, no. 11 (1992): 1165-69.

20◆. a. Suekawa, M., Ishige, A., Yuasa, K., Sudo, K., et al. "Pharmacological studies on ginger. I. Pharmacological actions of pungent constitutents, (6)-gingerol and (6)-shogaol." *Journal of Pharmacobio-dynamics* 7, no. 11 (Nov. 19894): 836-48.

b. Wu, H., Ye, D., Bai, Y., and Zhao, Y. ["Effect of dry ginger and roasted ginger on experimental gastric ulcers in rats."] *Chung-Kuo Chung Yao Tsa Chih [Ching Journal of Chinese Materia]* 15, no. 5 (May 1990): 278-80, 317-18.

21. Ye, D. J., Ding, A.W., and Guo, R. ["A research on the constituents of ginger in various preparations."] *Chung-Kuo Chung Yao Tsa Chih [China Journal of Chinese Materia]* 14, no. 5 (May 1989): 278-80, 318.

22. Govindarajan, V. S. "Ginger—Chemistry, technology, and quality evaluation: Part 2." *Critical Reviews in Food Science and Nutrition* 17, no. 3 (1982): 189-258 (p. 227).

23. Ibid., 221.

24. Heinerman, J., *Heinerman's Encyclopedia of Fruits, Vegetables and Herbs*, West Nyack, N.Y.: Parker, 1988, 154.

25. Cost, B. *Ginger: East to West.* Reading, Mass.: Addison-Wesley, 1989, 164.

26. Heinerman, J. *The Complete Book of Spices.* New Canaan, Conn.: Keats, 1983, 38-39.

27. a. Allen, K.L., Molan, P.C., and Reid, G.M. "A survey of the antibacterial activity of some New Zealand honeys." *Journal of Pharmacy and Pharmocology* 43, no. 12 (Dec. 1991): 817-22.

b. Jeddar, A., Kharsany, A., Ramsaroop, U.G., Bhamjee, A., et al. "The antibacterial action of honey. An in vitro study." *South African Medical Journal* 67, no. 7 (Feb. 1985): 257-58.

c. Willix, D. J., Molan, P. C., and Harfoot, C. G. "A comparison of the sensitivity of wound-infecting species of bacteria to the anti-bacterial activity of manuka honey and other honey." *Journal of Applied Bacteriology* 73, no. 5 (Nov. 1992): 388-94.

28. Gribel', N. V., and Pashinskii, V.G. ["The antitumor properties of honey."] *Voprosy Onkologii* 36, no. 6 (1990): 704-9.

29. a. Wellford, T. E., Eadie, T., and Llewellyn, G. C. "Evaluating the inhibitory action of honey on fungal growth, sporulation, and aflatoxin production." *Zeitschrift für Lebensmittel-untersuchung und Forschung* 166, no. 5 (June 1978): 280-83.

b. Obaseiki-Ebor, E. E., and Afonya, T. C. "In vitro evaluation of the anticandidiasis activity of honey distillate (HY-1) compared with that of some antimycotic agents." *Journal of Pharmacy and Pharmacology* 36, no. 4 (Apr. 1984): 283-84.

30. a. Efem, S. E., Udoh, K. T., and Iwara, C. I. "The antimicrobial spectrum of honey and its clinical significance." *Infection* 20, no. 4 (July-Aug. 1992): 227-29.

b. Ndayisaba, G., Bazira, L., Habonimana, E. ["Treatment of wounds with honey. 40 cases."] *Presse Medicale* 21, no. 32 (Oct. 1992): 1516-18.

c. Efem, S. E. "Clinical observations on the wound healing properties of honey." *British Journal of Surgery* 75, no. 7 (July 1988): 679-81.

d. Subrahmanyam, M. "Topical application of honey in treatment of burns." *British Journal of Surgery* 78, no. 4

(Apr. 1991): 497-98.

e. Bergman, A., Yanai, J., Weiss, J., Bell, D., and David, M. P. "Acceleration of wound healing by topical application of honey. An animal model." *American Journal of Surgery* 145, no. 3 (Mar. 1983): 374-76.

f. Efem, S. E. "Recent advances in the management of Fournier's gangrene: Preliminary observations." [see comments] *Surgery* 113, no. 2 (Feb. 1993): 200-204.

g. Phuapradit, W., and Saropala, N. "Topical application of honey in treatment of abdominal wound disruption." *Australian and New Zealand Journal of Obstetrics and Gynaecology* 32, no. 4 (Nov. 1992): 381-84.

31. a. Ali, A. T., Chowdhury, M.N., and Al Humayyd, M.S. "Inhibitory effect of natural honey on Helicobacter pylori." *Tropical Gastroenterology* 12, no. 3 (July-Sept. 1991): 139-43.

b. Ali, A. T. "Prevention of ethanol-induced gastric lesions in rats by natural honey, and its possible mechanism of action." *Scandinavian Journal of Gastroenterology* 26, no. 1 (Mar. 1991): 281-88.

c. Haffejee, I.E., and Moosa, A. "Honey in the treatment of infantile gastroenteritis." *British Medical Journal [Clinical Research Ed.]* 290, no. 6485 (June 1985): 1866-67.

32. See reference 31b.

33. Ali, A. T., Chowdhury, M.N., and Al Humayyd, M.S. "Inhibitory effect of natural honey on Helicobacter pylori." *Tropical*

Gastroenterology 12, no. 3 (July-Sept. 1991): 139-43.

34. a. Samanta, A., Burden, A. C., and Jones, G.R. "Plasma glucose responses to glucose, sucrose, and honey in patients with diabetes mellitus: An analysis of glycaemic and peak incremental indices." *Diabetic Medicine* 2, no. 5 (Sept. 1985): 371-73.

b. Bornet, F., Haardt, M. J., Costagliola, D., Blayo, A., and Slama, G. "Sucrose or honey at breakfast have no additional acute hyperglycaemic effect over an isoglucidic amount of bread in type 2 diabetic patients." *Diabetologia* 28, no. 4 (Apr. 1985): 213-17.

c. Shambaugh, P., Worthington, V., and Herbert, J. H. "Differential effects of honey, sucrose, and fructose on blood sugar levels." [see comments] *Journal of Manipulative and Physiological Therapeutics* 13, no. 6 (July-Aug. 1990): 322-25.

d. Akhtar, M. S., and Khan, M. S. "Glycaemic responses to three different honeys given to normal and alloxan-diabetic rabbits." *Jpma [Journal of the Pakistan Medical Association* 39, no. 4 (Apr. 1989): 107-13.

35. Obaseiki-Ebor, E. E., Afonya, T. C. "In-vitro evaluation of the anti-candidiasis activity of honey distillate (HY-1) compared with that of some antimycotic agents." *Journal of Pharmacy and Pharmacology* 36, no. 4 (Apr. 1984): 283-84.

36. See reference 26.

37. *Science News*, Biomedicine section, 25 Sept. 1993.

38. Govindarajan, V. S. "Ginger—

Chemistry, technology, and quality evaluation: Part 1." *Critical Reviews in Food Science and Nutrition* 17, no. 1 (1982): 1-96 (p. 53), citing Winterton, D., and Richardson, K. "An investigation into the chemical constituents of Queensland grown ginger." *Queensland Journal of Agricultural Sciences* 22 (1965): 205.

39. Lumb, A. B. "Effect of dried ginger on human platelet function." *Thrombosis and Haemostasis* 71, no. 1 (Jan. 1994): 110-1.

40. Srivastava, K. C., and Mustafa, T. "Ginger (*Zingiber officinale*) in rheumatism and musculoskeletal disorders." *Medical Hypotheses* 39, no. 4 (Dec. 1992): 342-48.

41. Fischer-Rasmussen, W., Kjaer, S. K., Dahl, C., and Asping, U. "Ginger treatment of hyperemesis gravidarum." *European Journal of Obstetrics, Gynecology, and Reproductive Biology* 38, no. 1 (Jan. 1991): 19-24.

42. See reference 40.

43. Personal communication with Julie Plunkett.

8. Freedom and Health at the Crossroads

1. Cynthia Cotts, *The Nation*, 31 Aug. – 7 Sept. 1992.

2. *Natural Health*, January/February 88.

3. Earthsave statistics from "How to Win an Argument with a Meat Eater."

4. National Research Council, 1982. "Diet, Nutrition, and Cancer." Washington, D.C.: National Academy Press, 55.

5. *Science News* 145 (1994): 102.

6. Kaiser Permanente Health Group, Longevity, June 1993.

7. Associated Press, *New York Times*, 26 May 1993.

8. Murray, M., 1991 SWHO Convention on Botanical Medicine.

9. Classen, D.C., et al. *JAMA* 226, no. 20 (Nov. 1991).

10. 1990 GAO (General Accounting Office) report, Washington, D.C.

11. Associated Press release, 22 Dec. 1992.

12. Little Rock Economic Conference, Associated Press release, 15 Dec. 1992.

13. Carter, J. A. *Racketeering in Medicine: The Suppression of Alternatives.* Hampton Roads: 1992.

14. AP release, November 1993

15. *New York Times*, 22 Sept. 1992.

16. a. See reference 10.

b. *New York Times*, 22 Sept. 1992.

c. Brody, J. "Vitamin E greatly reduces risk of heart disease. Studies suggest best results found in those taking large doses." *New York Times*, 20 May 1993.

17. a. Saito, Y., Kimura, Y., and Sakamoto, T. "The antioxidant effects of petroleum ether soluble and insoluble fractions from spices." *Eiyo to Shokuryo* 29 (1976): 505-10.

b. Huang, J., et al. "Studies on the antioxidative activities of spices grown in Taiwan." *Chung-Kuo Nung Yeh Hua Hsueh Hui Chih* 19, (1981): 3-4.

c. Lee, Chan Juan, et al.

"Studies on the antioxidative activities of spices grown in Taiwan." *Chemical Abstracts* 97, no. 3 (1982).

d. Toda, S., Kimura, M., et al. "Natural antioxidants antioxidative components isolated from schizandra fruit." *Shoyakugaku Zasshi* 42, no. 2 (1988): 156-59.

e. Shalini, V.K., and Srinivas, L. "Lipid peroxide induced DNA damage: Protection by turmeric (Curcuma longa)." *Mollecular and Cellular Biochemistry* 77 (1987): 3-10.

f. Walker, M. "Pycnogenol: Powerful antioxidant." *Natural Health*, July/August 1993, 40-41.

18. a. Plyasunova, O.A., Pokrovsky, A. G., Rusakov, I. A., Baltina, L. A., et al. "Inhibition of HIV reproduction in cell cultures by glycyrrhizic acid." *International Conference on AIDS* 8, no. 3 (July 19-24, 1992): 31.

b. Pliasunova, O. A., Egoricheva, I. N., Fediuk, N. V., Pokrovskii, A. G., et al. ["The anti-HIV activity of beta-glycyrrhizic acid."] *Voprosy Virusologii* 37, nos. 5-6 (Sept.-Dec. 1992): 235-38.

c. Shashikanth, K. N., Basappa, S. C., and Sreenivasa Murthy, V. "A comparative study of raw garlic extract and tetracycline on caecal microflora and serum proteins of albino rats." *Folia Microbiologica* (Praha) 29, no. 4 (1984): 348-52.

d. Russin, W. A., Hoesly, J. D., Elson, C. E., Tanner, M. A., and Gould, M. N. "Inhibition of rat mammary carcinogenesis by monoterpenoids." *Carcinogenesis* 10, no. 11 (Nov. 1989): 2161-64.

e. Elegbede, J. A., Elson, C. E., Qureshi, A., Tanner, M. A., and Gould, M. N. "Inhibition of DMBA-induced mammary cancer by the monoterpene d-limonene." *Carcinogenesis* 5, no. 5 (May 1984): 661-64.

f. Murray, M. T. *Natural Alternatives to Over-the-Counter and Prescription Drugs.* New York: Morrow, 1994, 383 pp.

19. *Larry King Live* (television show), aired 1992.

20. McCaleb, R. "Rational Regulation of Herbal Products Testimony before the Subcommittee on Government Regulations," citing Snider, S. "Beware the unknown brew; herbal teas and toxicity." *FDA Consumer* 25, no. 4 (1991): 30-33.

21. Ibid. citing *Innovations in Medicine #17*, Pharmaceutical Manufacturers' Association.

22. Annual Meeting, Federation of American Societies for Experimental Biology, New Orleans, La., 31 March 1993 (two other high officials confirmed).

23. 1990 GAO (General Accounting Office) report, Washington, D.C.

24. "Medical Controversy," *Time*, 18 March 1991.

25. *FDA Task Force Report*, Washington, D.C., 15 June 1993.

26. Associated Press release, Chicago, 12 May 1993.

27. Philip Holzberer, in editorial in *New York Times*, 7 Jan. 1993.

28. *Vegetarian Times*, February 1993.

29. Chren, M-M., and Landefeld, S. "Physicians' Behavior and Their Interactions with Drug Companies." *JAMA* 271 (1994): 684-89.

30. *Vegetarian Times*, May 1994, 22.

31. Associated Press release, *New York Times*, 2 Jan. 1993, 1.

32. Tierra, M. *American Herbalism.* Freedom, Calif.: Crossing Press. From essay by Jeanne Rose.

33. Heinerman, J. *The Science of Herbal Medicine.* Orem, Utah: Bi-World, 1979, 10.

Ginger's Constituents and Actions

1. Duke, J. A. *Phytochemical Constituents of GRAS Herbs and Other Economic Plants* (Database). CRC Press, 1992.

2. Duke, J. A. *Handbook of Biologically Active Phytochemicals and Their Activities.* CRC Press, 1992, 183 pp.

3. *Napralert Constituent Report*: Napralert Database, College of Pharmacy, University of Illinois.

4. Lawrence, B. "Major tropical spices — Ginger (*Zingiber officinale Rosc.*)." *Perfumer and Flavorist* 9 (Oct.–Nov. 1984): 35-36.

Appendix

ⓔⓒⓢⓠ

Resources

1. Naturopathy: Associations and Colleges

American Association of Naturopaths: For a list of practicing naturopathic physicians in your area, please send a self-addressed, stamped envelope to the Association (2366 East Lake Ave. E./ Suite 322/ Seattle, WA 98102).

COLLEGES OF NATUROPATHIC MEDICINE:

SW College of Naturopathic Medicine, 6535 E. Osborn Rd. #703/ Scottsdale, AZ 85251. Tel: 602/990-7424 (to be accredited)
Bastyr University of Naturopathic Medicine, 144 NE 54th Street/ Seattle, WA 98105. Tel: 206/523-9585
National College of Naturopathic Medicine, 11231 SE Market St./ Portland, OR 97216. Tel: 503/255-4860
Canadian College of Naturopathic Medicine, 60 Berl Ave./ Toronto, Ontario M8Y 3C7 Canada

2. Health Freedom Organizations

Citizens for Health, P.O. Box 1195, Tacoma, WA 98401. Tel: 206/922-2457

Nutritional Health Alliance, P.O. Box 267, Farmingdale, NY 11735. Tel: 800-226-4NHA

National Nutritional Foods Association, 125 E. Baker St., Ste. 230, Costa Mesa, CA 92626. Tel: 714/966-6632

3. Herbal Research Organizations

American Botanical Council, P.O. Box 201660, Austin, TX 78720. Tel: 512/331-8868

American Herbal Products Association, P.O. Box 2410, Austin, TX 78768. Tel: 512/320-8555

American Herbalists Guild, P.O. Box 1683, Soquel, CA 95073. Tel: 408/464-2441

Herb Research Foundation, 1007 Pearl St., Ste. 200, Boulder, CO 80302. Tel: 303/449-2265

Recommended Reading

Rudolph Ballentine, M.D. *Diet and Nutrition*. Honesdale, Pa.: The Himalayan International Institute of Yoga Science and Philosophy, 1978.

Deepak Chopra, M.D. *Quantum Healing*. New York: Bantam, 1989.

Dr. John R. Christopher. *School of Natural Healing*. Provo, Utah: BiWorld Publishers, 1976.

Larry Dossey, M.D. *Meaning and Medicine*. New York: Bantam, 1992

Rosemary Gladstar. *Herbal Healing for Women*. New York: Simon & Schuster, 1993.

Barbara Griggs. *Green Pharmacy*. Rochester, Vt.: Healing Arts Press, 1981.

Jethro Kloss. *Back to Eden*. Santa Barbara, Calif.: Woodbridge Press Publishing Co., 93111.

Dr. Vasant Lad and David Frawley. *The Yoga of Herbs*. Santa Fe: Lotus Press, 1986.

John A. McDougall, M.D. *McDougall's Medicine*. Piscataway, N.J.: New Century Publishers, 1985.

Daniel B. Mowrey, Ph.D. *The Scientific Validation of Herbal Medicine*. Cormorant Books, 1986.

Michael T. Murray, N.D. *Natural Alternatives to Over-the-Counter and Prescription Drugs.* New York: Morrow, 1994.

Michael T. Murray, N.D., and Joseph Pizzorno, N.D. *Encyclopedia of Natural Medicine.* Rocklin, Calif.: Prima Publishing, 1991.

Thomas A. Newmark, and Paul Schulick *Beyond Aspirin: Nature's Challenge To Arthritis, Cancer & Alzheimer's Disease.* Prescott, Az.: Hohm Press, 2000.

Dean Ornish, M.D. *Dr. Dean Ornish's Program for Reversing Heart Disease.* New York: Ballantine, 1990.

John Robbins. *Diet for a New America.* Walpole, N. H.: Stillpoint Publishing, 1987.

Ron Teeguarden. *Chinese Tonic Herbs.* Tokyo and New York: Japan Publications, 1984.

Dr. H. C. A. Vogel. *The Nature Doctor.* New Canaan, Conn.: Keats Publishing, 1952.

Andrew Weil, M.D. *Natural Health, Natural Medicine.* Boston: Houghton Mifflin, 1990.

Rudolf Fritz Weiss, M.D. *Herbal Medicine.* Stuttgart, Germany: Hippokrates Verlag, 1988 (distributor: Medicina Biologica, Portland, Oreg.).

Index

❧❦❧❦

A

abortion, 18, 105
adaptogenic, 16 53, 54, 105
alcohol, 29, 40, 59, 77, 81-82
analgesic, 16, 75, 102, 105
Anisakis, 47, 48
anthelmintic, 14, 15, 16, 47, 48, 75, 105
anti-inflammatory, 14, 15, 16, 18, 19, 30, 31, 32, 33, 38, 45, 50, 52, 57, 64, 75, 80, 81, 103, 105
anti-aggregatory, 36, 45
antiarthritic, 102
antibacterial, 14, 15, 50, 78, 80, 105
antibiotics, 15, 27
antiemetic, 43
antifungal, 29, 50, 78, 80, 105
antihistaminic, 50
antimicrobial, 28, 42, 102
antimutagenic, 51, 103, 105
antioxidant, 14, 16, 58, 66, 92, 93, 102, 106
antiparasitic, 102, 103
antithrombic, 106
antitussive, 16, 50, 80, 106
antiulcer, 41, 58, 78, 87, 103
antiviral, 50, 106
aphrodisiac, 25, 26, 28, 29, 54, 103, 106
aromatherapeutic, 81
arthritis, 13, 17, 27, 31, 32, 33,34, 50, 65, 86, 88, 103
Ascaris, 47, 48, 49
aspirin, 18, 19, 33, 34, 35, 36, 37, 52, 57, 59, 64, 81, 85, 103

asthma, 28, 30, 32, 77, 79
Ayurvedic, 23, 46, 50, 78

B

Backon, Joshua, 54, 57, 84, 87
benzo(a)pyrene, 103
BHA, 36
BHT, 36
bioavailability, 16, 46, 54, 77, 86, 103, 106
blood pressure, 35, 45, 54
blood sugar, 54, 78, 104
botany, 5
breech births, 54
Brody, Jane, 47

C

caffeic esters, 80
cancer, 19, 35, 36, 51, 52, 78, 80, 90, 92, 97, 103, 104, 105, 107
candida albicans, 78
cardiovascular, 18, 34, 36, 37, 81, 86, 103
carminative, 28, 29, 30, 106
carrot juice, 77
chemotherapy, 43
chills, 37
chlorinated hydrocarbons, 72
cholesterol, 54
cimetidine, 39, 40, 67
circulatory, 30, 34, 35, 52, 53, 54, 62, 84, 104
clogged arteries, 35
cold remedy, 29, 76, 103

About the Author

Paul Schulick is an herbalist and advocate of personal choice in health care. A comprehensive library of herbal texts and a collection of international medical databases support the author's theories and tradition-based herbal formulations. His research extends from the therapeutic values of plants harvested from the seas to the healing powers of herbs commonly found in the spice cabinet. The author lectures throughout the country on the health impact of herbs and natural foods.

Paul lives and works with his wife, Barbi, and their children, Geremy and Rosalie, in Brattleboro, Vermont.